The Sphincter of Oddi Dysfunction Survival Guide

The Ultimate Resource for Diagnosis, Treatment, and Living Well with SOD

By Brooke Keefer

Table of Contents

Copyright and Disclaimer 1
Dedication and Acknowledgments 2
Introduction 3
Chapter 1: My Story 6
Chapter 2: What is SOD? 16
Chapter 3: Causes of SOD 26
Chapter 4: Finding an SOD Doctor 40
Chapter 5: Diagnostic Tests 50
Chapter 6: Natural Treatments 63
Chapter 7: SOD Diet 80
Chapter 8: Medications 89
Chapter 9: Procedural and Surgical Treatments 101
Chapter 10: Self-Care and Support 119
Chapter 11: Emergency Rooms and Hospitals 135
Chapter 12: Be an Empowered Patient 144
Chapter 13: If It Isn't SOD What Is Wrong with Me? 152
Chapter 14: The Future of SOD 159
Closing Statement 176
Bibliography 177
About the Author 182

Copyright and Disclaimer

1st Edition

© 2016 Brooke Keefer – All Rights Reserved

No part of this publication may be reproduced, stored in a retrieval system or transmitted in any form or by any means electronic, mechanical or otherwise, without permission of the publisher of this book.

All material in this book is provided for your information only and may not be construed as medical advice or instruction. No action or inaction should be taken based solely on the contents of this information; instead, readers should consult appropriate health professionals on any matter relating to their health and well-being.

The information and opinions expressed here are believed to be accurate, based on the best judgment available to the author, and readers who fail to consult with appropriate health professionals assume the risk of any injuries. In addition, the information and opinions expressed here do not necessarily reflect the views of every contributor to the book. The author acknowledges occasional differences in opinion and welcomes the exchange of different viewpoints. The publisher is not responsible for errors or omissions.

Readers interested in sending their suggestions, ideas or comments can do so via email at info@sodae.org or visit www.sodae.org.

Dedication and Acknowledgments

This book is dedicated to sphincter of Oddi dysfunction patients, their families, caregivers, and friends. May this book help bring wellness back into your lives. This is as much your book as it is mine.

I would like to pay special thanks to my family, especially my mother (Linda), father (Donald), stepmother (Janice), stepfather (John), husband (Bill), and children (Alex, Schyler, Ashley, Andrew, and William). Your love, patience, and concern was beyond anything I could have imagined. Even as sick as I was I always felt loved and supported.

Thank you to my dear friends who put up with my moaning and groaning day and night. I got through many horrible times because of your support.

Much gratitude to Joe and everyone at Policy Research Associates for being such an outstanding and compassionate employer. And, though I complain about the medical profession throughout this book, I must point out and acknowledge the doctors who didn't give up on me and showed compassion, namely Dr. Francois Vachon, Dr. Martin Freeman, Dr. Joseph Bell, Dr. Abdelhakim Dinar, Dr. Sven Hida, Dr. Jose Posada, and Dr. Ankesh Nigam.

Introduction

I decided to write this book as there were few patient-friendly resources on sphincter of Oddi dysfunction (SOD). I searched high and low for information and the only book about SOD I found was a textbook written in 1976. I could not even locate a brochure on SOD. All of the information I did happen to find on the Internet was written in research or medical jargon. Luckily, I am fairly intelligent and could decipher the big words and confusing lingo. However, I often thought how terrible it must be for patients having difficulty interpreting it all, who were desperate for information about their condition.

I discovered the most helpful SOD information out there did not exist on a website or in a book. It did not come from my doctors either. The best information I gathered on SOD was from fellow SOD sufferers. Without my experience participating in Internet SOD support groups, I would not have gathered half the information I am about to share with you.

This guide is a compendium of my and other SOD patients' personal experiences with trying to find a diagnosis, obtain treatment, and develop coping strategies. I also included a good amount of information regarding the science behind SOD, which I tried my best to decipher into laymen's terms. Of course, in some cases, it was impossible to not use research and medical lingo to describe aspects of this condition. SOD is complex. It is a complicated condition in a complicated area of the body.

I hope you can get what you need from this book and "leave the rest." Some of you may only want to read the chapters on diagnosis and treatments, while others will be quite interested in the science behind SOD. Even if the scientific content does not appeal to you, I encourage you to read it. I think it is important people understand why their bodies are sick, as it can help lead them to recovery. It is empowering to have information about the condition affecting your life. Whatever brought you here to read this book, I can promise you that as of this writing it is the most thorough, patient-driven resource about SOD out there.

The goal of this guide is for SOD sufferers, their families, and friends to gain a better understanding of this elusive disease and find effective ways to achieve wellness despite dealing with often-times multiple symptoms. I hope physicians and natural health care practitioners read this book as well. In fact, encourage your doctors to read it. Many doctors are left stumped on how to help their SOD patients find relief and could learn ways to not only treat their patients but to support them too. Natural health practitioners can be particularly helpful for SOD patients, but often know very little about SOD. I had to educate every natural health practitioner that treated me. This was essential so they could effectively treat me.

You may wonder what qualifies me to write this book. I do not have a medical degree (hence no M.D. at the end of my name), Ph.D., natural health degree, or any kind of healthcare degree. I have a Bachelor of Arts degree in Mathematics and much of my career over the past 15-years has been in the field of children's mental health and juvenile justice advocacy and reform.

I have no formal training in anything to do with the gastrointestinal system. That being said, I have no problem saying I am an SOD expert of sorts. I am a 17-year survivor of SOD. Thirty-five percent of my life here on Earth has been spent living with SOD. I have tried the majority of treatments, procedures, and surgeries mentioned in this book. I have lived with mild SOD and full-blown disabling SOD. I have read any and all research on SOD I could find on the Internet, especially the National Institutes of Health's PubMed website. I have done so much health research since getting sick with SOD that I get every answer correct when there is a medical category on the television show Jeopardy.

In 2012, I started The Sphincter of Oddi Dysfunction Awareness and Education Network (The SODAE Network), a not for profit organization with its own website (www.sodae.org); and its own Facebook page (https://www.facebook.com/sphincterofoddi)) and

Facebook support group (https://www.facebook.com/groups/SODAE). My active participation in numerous Internet support groups for SOD, chronic pancreatitis, IBS, gastroparesis, IBS and other digestive disorders has educated me greatly. Peer to peer support and education has been the cornerstone of my recovery and the source of vital SOD information. I pay attention and learn from others. I have lived and breathed this cruddy disease with every breath of my being and this guide is a testament to all I have learned along the way.

The only thing I don't have experience in is medically treating SOD patients. Therefore, I must tell you that all of the information contained in this book is for informational purposes only. In no way am I intending to diagnose or treat any person's condition. That is the job of a doctor or other healthcare professional. Use this information as a tool and not a prescription. Always consult with your doctors about introducing a treatment or removing a treatment. Do not self-medicate even natural remedies like supplements and herbs. They can be contraindicated for your condition or interact with medications you are taking.

Remember as you read this book that my story is a worst case scenario of sorts. Do not think everything I experienced will happen to you or the person you know with SOD. My SOD was very manageable for a long time. It was not always horrible. Remain positive and remember while reading this guide you are unique. Just as every stroke, cancer, diabetes and heart disease patient is different, so is every SOD patient. There are different types and stages of SOD. Symptoms vary as well. You are more likely to recover and live a quality life than end up an extreme case like I became. Hopefully, in utilizing the information you are about to read, you will prevent a worst case scenario from happening or learn to get through your own version of a worst case scenario.

Whatever the situation or case, I hope this book helps you. I wish you total wellness on your SOD journey. Never ever give up!

Chapter 1: My Story

In 1998, I had my gallbladder removed. Within a few weeks, I developed a sharp pain in my right side under my ribs that radiated to my back and shoulder. This was vastly different from my gallbladder pain, which had been more of a dull ache around my sternum. I also had nausea and a constant "full" feeling which the gallbladder removal seemed to have cured. Since this new right side pain was quickly becoming debilitating, my primary care and gastrointestinal (GI) doctors ordered an endoscopy, barium enema, and blood work.

All tests came back normal. My GI doctor said I must have Irritable Bowel Syndrome (IBS) and to drink Metamucil. He also entered me into a clinical trial for an antispasmodic medication, which, due to the side effects, I had to discontinue. I was discouraged but trusted my doctor's diagnosis.

For the next 13 years, I learned to live with the pain, accepting IBS as my diagnosis. The first year was the worst. The pain was relentless. I cried and moaned day and night. Even so, I refused to take narcotic pain medication, which actually ended up being a good thing as some opioid drugs are known to cause SOD spasms. Instead, I focused on deep breathing exercises, yoga, and a low-fat diet to ease the pain.

Fortunately, as time went on, the pain lessened and became more of an annoyance than a debilitating condition. Yes, the pain was always there and I had flare ups, but I was constantly learning about ways to cope and live with it. I can honestly say I was able to have a quality life. I was successful in my career, traveling the United States as a children's mental health advocate. I enjoyed my family and raised my boys.

Fast forward to September 2, 2011. Three months after delivering my third son by C-section, I became suddenly and severely ill with no appetite, dizziness, brain fog, fatigue, vomiting, and abdominal pain that spread to the area under my sternum. It is important to note that during this pregnancy my constant right side pain magically disappeared. I didn't think there was a connection with these new symptoms. I figured my symptoms had something to do with the antibiotic I was taking for a bad bout of mastitis. I had developed an infected milk duct from breastfeeding.

A visit to the emergency room on September 5, 2011, proved to be uneventful. All of my blood work came back normal, as did my stool sample. My symptoms did not improve and an endoscopy a few weeks later showed only mild gastritis and large amounts of bile collecting in my stomach, but nothing else.

On September 21, 2011, nine days before my 42nd birthday, I was hospitalized for dehydration, vomiting, and abdominal pain that I rated as a 9 on the 1 to 10 pain scale. I was admitted to the hospital for five days and given a healthy dose of intravenous fluids, anti-anxiety, anti-nausea, and pain medication. They also tried me on what I nicknamed a "munchy-inducing" anti-depressant, called Remeron (mirtazapine) because I think they thought I had an eating disorder.

It truly did give me the "munchies" but the problem was that eating was not the problem. Digestion was the issue. I had a CT scan, which was normal, as was my blood work. Prior to being discharged on five or six different medications, the GI doctor who performed the endoscopy told my dad he thought my symptoms were caused by post-partum depression. Basically, the doctor was saying this was all in my head.

My family and I knew otherwise so I sought out a second opinion from another GI group. I thought the new GI doctor would be compassionate as she was a woman. She performed a colonoscopy, though I hadn't had bowel symptoms in a month. It was a waste of a copay, a waste of one of many copays. This female doctor was the exact opposite of compassionate. She spent two minutes with me after the procedure to tell me my colonoscopy was normal except for a few hemorrhoids.

Then she told me I needed to be on an antidepressant as she thought my condition was psychological. I told her if she read my chart she would have seen I was already on an antidepressant. No sooner did I say that than she left my bedside to talk to another patient. I sobbed, feeling helpless and hopeless. Here was another doctor who thought my condition was all in my head.

This led me to a third opinion with a well-respected, local surgeon. This was the first time sphincter of Oddi dysfunction (SOD) was introduced to my vocabulary. He felt it was a strong possibility I had SOD, but first wanted to rule out any vascular issues so off I was to get a CT Angiogram scan of my abdomen. This test showed veins and arteries and of course it came back normal. The surgeon told me verbally and in writing that he strongly suspected I had SOD and should be tested for it.

He explained the "gold standard" diagnostic test for SOD was an endoscopic retrograde cholangiopancreatography (ERCP) with sphincter of Oddi manometry. I will explain this ridiculously long medical term later on, but in a nutshell this type of ERCP is an endoscopic procedure down the throat that utilizes x-rays to gather images of the biliary and pancreatic ducts (drainage routes) of the gallbladder, liver, and pancreas and obtain pressures of the biliary, pancreatic and oddi sphincters.

Since my original GI doctors—the first local GI practice I visited—were the only doctors who performed this type of ERCP in my hometown, the surgeon personally called the practice to (strongly) recommend I get this very specialized test. "Great," I thought, "I will get my diagnosis and get treatment."

Not so fast. I would have to wait another two months to get an appointment with the local GI doctor who specialized in pancreatic/biliary issues. He was in the same practice as the original GI doctor. I know, it is very confusing. As a consolation, I even have difficulty getting the doctors straight because I have seen so many—around ten different GI doctors since my SOD journey began.

The reason it took two months to see this specialist was because the GI practice made me see my original GI doctor first before I could see the actual SOD specialist—it was the practice's policy. It made no sense other than for the practice to make an extra buck having me waste my time with the original guy before I could get in with the real expert. In his defense, he did make one last ditch effort to help me by prescribing antispasmodics. None helped and the side effects ended up being intolerable.

I continued to have symptoms and was losing weight at an alarming rate. Shortly after this visit, I was hospitalized for four days right before Christmas for nausea, vomiting, dehydration, and pain. There, I had an upper GI series (a scan where I swallowed radioactive liquid as an x-ray traced how the liquid flowed through my upper digestive system) and more blood work, which were—you guessed it—normal.

Somehow, through all of this, I was pushing myself to show up for work and be a mom to my infant and teenage son, while existing (I wouldn't call it living) with these disabling symptoms. I woke up puking, weak, in pain and pretty much felt that way all day and night. The best part of my day was going to sleep to get a reprieve from the horrible symptoms.

I saw the "new" GI doctor from the same practice in January 2012. He suspected something was going on with my pancreas from the way I described my abdominal pain. He trialed me on prescription pancreatic enzymes (Creon), which, after a week, brought the searing pain under my sternum from a constant 7 out of 10 to a manageable 3 or 4 out of 10 (as long as I took them with every meal and snack). The enzyme copays were expensive and my husband and I were going broke from prescription, inpatient, procedural, and office visit copays. Weight was flying off of my petite frame. I was becoming skin and bones, a shell of a person. If I hadn't been "crazy" by now as my doctors thought, I'd be crazy for not being crazy!

The specialist thought I had chronic pancreatitis (CP), so instead of doing the ERCP, he performed an endoscopic ultrasound (EUS) on February 14, 2012. I was furious as I wanted the ERCP with manometry so I could be tested for SOD, which would also test for CP, basically killing two birds with one stone. The EUS showed a healthy pancreas—another normal test. The doctor told me he wouldn't do an ERCP to test for SOD mainly because even if I had SOD, he didn't see much success in the treatments and that a national study was showing poor results of invasive treatments.

Fed up and desperate, I searched the Internet for other people like me who had similar SOD symptoms. I found an old blog where several people recommended a physician located in Minneapolis, Minnesota. Though I lived in upstate New York, I scheduled an appointment with him. Fortunately, my insurance covered the medical expenses, minus copays and travel. Unfortunately, the wait to see him was three months out. I took the appointment anyways. I sure as heck wasn't getting any help locally.

In April 2012, I saw the local GI specialist one last time. He entered the exam room and said, "Oh dear. You look anorexic." He told me to reduce the stress in my life and to eat more. Uh duh. If I could eat more I would. Again, he refused to perform the ERCP and pretty much put the blame on me for why I was so ill and emaciated and pretty much threatened me that I'd soon need a feeding tube. The feeding tube threat actually sounded wonderful considering how awful eating made me feel. At this point, I was down to 100 pounds from the 135 pounds I weighed before getting sick. I hadn't weighed 100 pounds since I was 14 years old! I felt weak, depressed, lost and hopeless.

By May 2012, I was 95 pounds and experiencing orthostatic hypotension where my blood pressure dropped dangerously low when I'd rise from lying or sitting down. This caused a few scary fainting spells. I was dizzy much of the time, had the usual 24/7 nausea, my muscles were wasting away, and as an added bonus I was losing my cognitive abilities. I had to leave my career as I was now severely disabled.

I looked like a victim of starvation and avoided mirrors and anyone with a camera. I could not gain or sustain weight on my own. On May 7, 2012, I flew with my mom to see the GI specialist in Minnesota. He was amazing. I cried over the fact I finally found a doctor who treated me with compassion and believed my illness was not a mental defect. He listened to me and genuinely wanted to help me get better. It was enlightening. It was the first time through all of this that I had a shred of hope.

He told me I likely had SOD and wanted to perform the ERCP test. However, I was so emaciated at this point that an ERCP could have killed me. Acute pancreatitis, a life-threatening condition, occurs in small percentages of people after this procedure. While I was in Minnesota, he had an associate perform another EUS and pancreatic functioning test. Both were fairly normal, except my bile duct was dilated and pancreatic duct had scarring.

Finally, something showed up on a test! Most people pray nothing shows up on a medical test. I, on the other hand, was elated. The specialist recommended in writing that I get a G/J feeding tube to bulk me up so I could return to Minnesota in August, which would be in two months, to have the ERCP with manometry performed.

Upon my return back home, and after going through a very difficult time trying to convince anyone to put the feeding tube in, I had a G-J feeding tube inserted on May 25, 2012. I began formula feeds internally through the J-tube. I was able to eat a minimal amount of food, about 700-800 calories. The tube became a whole other set of issues. The J part that was supposed to stay in the small intestine kept migrating into my duodenum (first part of the small intestine) and stomach, defeating the whole purpose of having a feeding tube as it bypassed the sphincter of Oddi area. I was nauseous all of the time—worse than ever. I had to be hospitalized to have my tube replaced five times in two months.

Also, the first few formula choices were not agreeing with me. I'd get severe nausea and headaches from them. It took over a month to find the right one. Through my own investigation, I realized I had a major sensitivity to formula containing casein protein, hence the headaches. Also, I later discovered I had fructose intolerance, which was a huge problem as the formulas were high in sugar and fructose. Gaining weight became a difficult full-time job.

By August I was able to get up to 109 pounds and flew back to Minnesota to have the ERCP. No surprise to anyone close to me, I was diagnosed with SOD. Beyond a shadow of a doubt, I had likely been suffering from SOD dating back to after my gallbladder removal. Basal pressures of the sphincters are supposed to be less than 35-40 mm/hg.

Mine were over 175 mm/hg. Most of the people I've met with SOD have pressures between 60 and 100 mm/hg. After determining I had SOD, the specialist performed a dual sphincterotomy (cutting) of my pancreatic and biliary sphincters to try and remedy my symptoms. Temporary stents were also placed in my bile and pancreatic ducts.

By now my mom had given me the nickname of "Murphy" because like Murphy's Law if anything could go wrong it did. In true Murphy form, I was one of the unlucky few who ended up with acute pancreatitis after the procedure. I also developed an E-coli blood infection that went septic. The diarrhea was unlike anything I ever experienced. It gushed out of me uncontrollably. Those poor nurses couldn't leave my side as I couldn't stop soiling myself and the linens. The acute pancreatic pain and nausea were unbearable too. I vomited, crapped, and felt like I was going to die for sure.

The doctors could not explain how I got an E-coli infection. We naturally have E-coli in our large bowels, not way up in our bile ducts. Recently, there have been news reports that ERCP scopes are to blame for superbug infections like this because they weren't sterilized properly. Regardless of how I got it, I am lucky to be alive. In fact, a darling resident physician at the hospital had to tell my mom, in front of me, that there was a good chance I wouldn't make it. All I kept thinking was I couldn't die in Minnesota and I had to get back to my husband and kids.

After a week in the hospital, four days of which were in the intensive care unit (ICU), I was discharged and flew home. No sooner did I get home than my feeding tube was kinked and had to be replaced at the local hospital. Just my luck. However, I was grateful to be alive and found slight relief from my SOD symptoms for about four weeks. Unfortunately, the relief was short-lived. A month after my near death experience, I ended up in the hospital yet again due to pain and nausea and to have my temporary stents removed. By now I switched hospitals and was going to the major medical center nearby, which was also a teaching hospital.

There, I met a very nice surgeon who suggested a more permanent solution—a transduodenal sphincteroplasty. He explained he could sew the sphincters permanently open to the duodenum. I was desperate at this point as I was back down to under 100 pounds and not functioning well. It was major surgery, but I knew I had to go for it, as I couldn't imagine living life so ill all the time.

On October 3, 2012, I had open abdominal surgery for the sphincteroplasty. It was major surgery and seemed to open the floodgates of bile. I had a drain but it only collected so much. The rest came out as bile diarrhea. My surgeon said he never saw it so bad as in me. Then, just when I thought I could be discharged I developed a life-threatening bacterial infection that went septic. This one was an Enterobacter strain. Possibly I got it from the ERCP I had in Albany to remove the stents. I will never really know for sure. This infection was even more deadly. I had a temperature hovering around 106 degrees and was violently shaking from rigors. I came very close to dying again. Only 50% of people survive sepsis. I survived it twice!

Because of this and other complications, I spent an entire month in the hospital. I was blessed to have not only a great surgeon but also a very compassionate one. In addition, the residents, my new local GI doctor (the fourth local GI), and nutritional MD, all treated me with respect and validated my condition rather than blaming and shaming me as my original doctors had done.

The recovery from the sphincteroplasty was a long one and took a lot of patience before I started feeling better. Some days I thought I would never be right. After a few months, my SOD seemed to heal, not fully but enough to feel "well." The 24/7 nausea was nearly gone and the pain was better. Tragically I wasn't well in other areas. I was given massive amounts of an antibiotic called Levaquin and steroids for the most recent sepsis incident. I had already been on a benzodiazepine, clonazepam (generic for Klonopin). Since steroids and benzodiazepines are contraindicated with fluoroquinolone antibiotics like Levaquin, it caused a poisonous reaction throughout my entire body, damaging tendons and my nervous system. I also had signs of mitochondrial damage.

Now there are all kinds of Food and Drug Administration (FDA) warnings about fluoroquinolone antibiotics like Levaquin, Cipro, and Avelox. Murphy strikes again. I got one problem "fixed" only to be left severely disabled by an antibiotic. The FDA calls it "fluoroquinolone associated disability." Those of us unlucky enough to have this affliction call it "fluoroquinolone toxicity syndrome." I am still recovering from essentially being poisoned, but I am better.

Last year I was diagnosed with chronic pancreatitis. I believe it coincided with coming off of that low dose benzodiazepine. It seems the withdrawal syndrome involved with these medications causes issues with parts of your body you are most vulnerable. I've met others like me and performed some testing of adding it back and withdrawing it again. Each time proved disastrous to my pancreas. I have calcifications and more scarring in my pancreas and duct. It is just a theory as nearly all of the SOD patients I know who had the sphincteroplasty surgery now have chronic pancreatitis, which has led me to believe those of us most difficult-to-treat SOD patients have severe issues with our pancreatic sphincter.

For the most part, though, I am doing quite well. I have a positive outlook most days. Thanks to caring doctors and treatments I have a quality of life. I watch what I eat, do yoga and meditation, see a therapist for the health-related mental health issues, run the www.sodae.org and www.haveahealthygut.com website and the

SODAE Network Facebook page and group write articles mostly on digestive issues, and spend as much time as I can with my family. I am truly blessed to have made it through this ordeal. Now it is my turn to give back and help anyone struggling with SOD.

SOD can be a debilitating disease that should be taken seriously by the healthcare profession as evidenced by my story. I can't imagine what my life would be like if I'd never gone to Minnesota or had major surgery. I honestly think I wouldn't be alive if I'd stuck it out with those local GI doctors. I hope by telling my story it will help someone get the help they need and know they are not alone and that SOD is not "in their head." There is really no sure-fire cure for SOD. However, it can be arrested with natural treatments, medications, procedures, or surgeries.

As I mentioned in the Introduction, my story is a worst case scenario for sure. Keep in mind, that I successfully lived with SOD for around 13 years before things went completely south. Something significant triggered the SOD into overdrive. Possibly it was childbirth and the subsequent fluctuation in hormones. Maybe it was the mastitis infection or the antibiotic for the infection. I will never know for certain. The point is to read this book and believe you will be ok because you will be armed with resources. Stay hopeful and determined.

Chapter 2: What is SOD?

Sphincter of Oddi dysfunction (SOD) is not easily explained by its title, nor is one definition agreed upon in scientific circles. Not only is sphincter of Oddi dysfunction eight syllables of complicated-sounding mumbo jumbo, numerous theories on what exactly *is* SOD abound. Ours is not a commonly understood disease like diabetes, celiac disease or diarrhea-predominant irritable bowel syndrome (IBS-D). If someone tells you they have diabetes, you know they have issues maintaining blood sugar levels. People with celiac have to avoid gluten, mostly wheat products. IBS-D is, well, self-explanatory. We visualize sufferers spending a lot of time in the bathroom.

When I tell people I have SOD, there is always a look the other person gives me as though they want to ask, "What the heck is that?" I try to explain SOD as simply and concisely as I can. I say something like, "It is a rare disease where the biliary and pancreatic sphincters don't work properly or they spasm shut." Afterward, that look of "What the heck is that?" turns into a look of "Aha. I think I can picture that happening."

Most people seem to understand what I am talking about, or at least they act like they do. Maybe they are just appeasing me. I do know for certain that nearly everyone I have educated on my condition never knew they had these sphincters that could wreak such havoc on someone's health and wellbeing. I went my entire life not knowing about these sphincters until one doctor suspected they were the cause of my disabling symptoms.

SOD Anatomy

To this day I do not fully understand the anatomy associated with SOD, but at least I am not alone. There is still much to be discovered regarding the sphincter of Oddi, especially how hormonal, endocrine and other bodily substances and functions affect this area of the body.

Sphincter of Oddi was named after the Italian physiologist, Ruggero Oddi, who discovered this area of the body in the late 1800s. Apparently, Ruggero Oddi was not the original discoverer of the sphincter. An English physician named Francis Glisson identified it two centuries earlier. Oddi was the first to distinguish the sphincters' physiological properties.

Johns Hopkins Hospital's website described SOD as follows:

Sphincter of Oddi dysfunction is a result of anatomic and physiologic abnormalities in the distal choledochus and sphincter. A variable length of the distal choledochus and the pancreatic duct are invested with circular and longitudinal smooth muscle fibers that interdigitate with the extra-ampullary muscle fibers of the duodenal wall to form the sphincter of Oddi. Mini sphincters, or three discrete areas of muscle thickness (sphincter papillae, sphincter pancreaticus, and sphincter choledochus), comprise the sphincter of Oddi. Upon ingestion of food, the gallbladder contracts, with a simultaneous decrease in the resistance in the sphincter of Oddi zone.

See why I am confused? What the heck did all that mean? Hopefully, I can decipher as best I can in laymen's terms.

SOD is a result of abnormalities in the bile duct and sphincter. There are a whole lot of muscle fibers in and around the biliary and pancreatic ducts. SOD is concerned mostly with those smooth muscle fibers around the entrance to these ducts, which is known as the ampulla of Vater. They run side to side and in a circular pattern. The sphincter of Oddi makes up all of these muscle fibers. Within this are three separate sphincters—the biliary, pancreatic, and main papillary (at the ampulla of Vater entrance connecting the duodenal section of the small intestine to the biliary and pancreatic ducts). Therefore, the sphincter of Oddi isn't just the sphincter, it is the entire smooth muscle that surrounds the end portion of the common bile and pancreatic ducts.

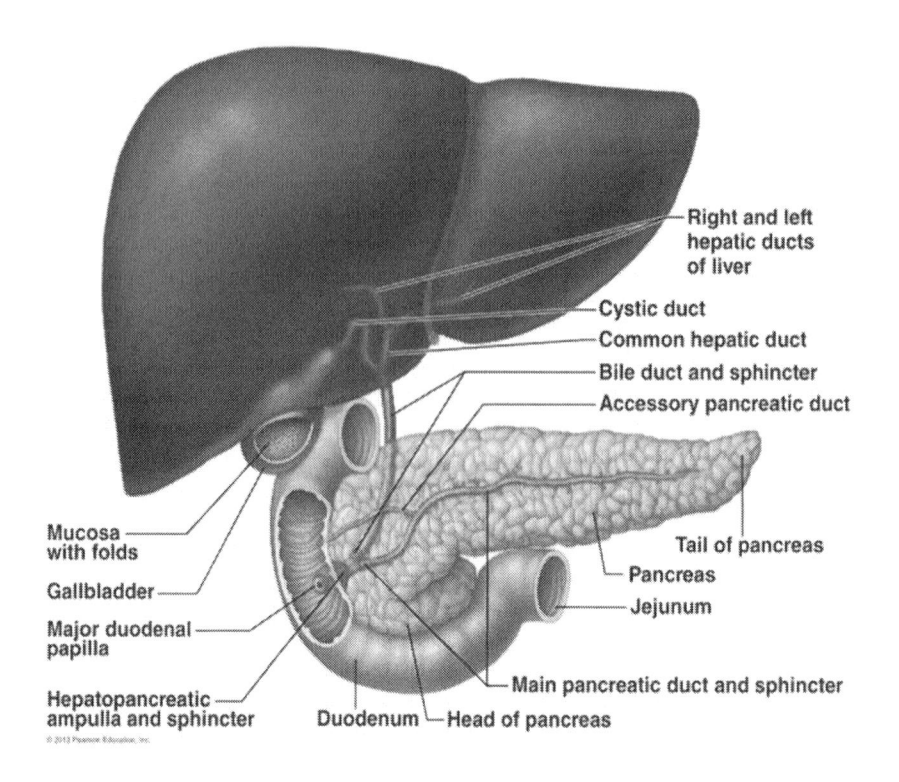

The primary purpose of the sphincters is to regulate the flow of bile and pancreatic juices. This muscle relaxes (opens) during a meal to allow bile and pancreatic juice to flow into the intestine. The sphincter controls the flow of bile and pancreatic juices into the duodenum (the first part of the small intestine in which the stomach drains) and prevents reflux of duodenal contents into the ducts.

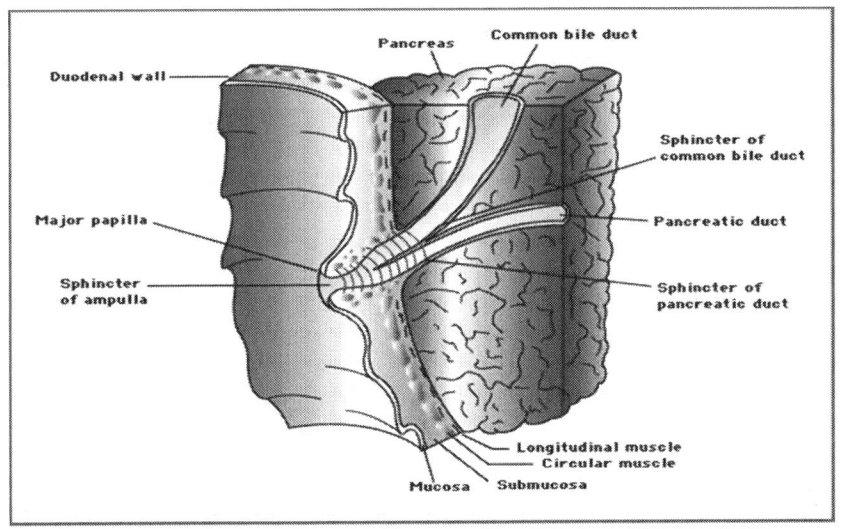

Sphincter of Oddi in relation to the ampulla of Vater Diagram of the anatomy of the sphincter of Oddi and ampulla of Vater. The muscle fibers of the sphincter of Oddi surround the intraduodenal segment of the common bile duct and the ampulla of Vater. A circular aggregate of muscle fibers, known as the sphincter choledochus (or sphincter of Boyden), keeps resistance to bile flow high, and thereby permits filling of the gallbladder during fasting and prevents retrograde reflux of duodenal contents into the biliary tree. A separate short structure, called the sphincter pancreaticus, encircles the distal pancreatic duct. The muscle fibers of the sphincter pancreaticus are interlocked with those of the sphincter choledochus in a figure eight pattern.

It has been proposed SOD is comprised of two pathologic entities:

Sphincter of Oddi stenosis (a mechanical abnormality): Sphincter of Oddi stenosis refers to a structural alteration of the sphincter, probably from an inflammatory process with subsequent fibrosis (scarring and thickening of tissue). In this case, papillary stenosis, a fixed anatomic narrowing of the sphincter often due to fibrosis, would be an example of sphincter of Oddi stenosis.

Sphincter of Oddi dyskinesia (a functional or motility abnormality): Sphincter of Oddi dyskinesia refers to a variety of pressure abnormalities and motor abnormalities of the sphincter of Oddi. These abnormalities may result in a hypotonic (slow acting) sphincter but more commonly, a hypertonic (overactive) sphincter. In a nutshell, the sphincter fails to relax properly.

The Three Types of SOD

Currently, physicians categorize SOD into three diagnostic categories or "Types" based on the Milwaukee classification system or Rome III criteria. All SOD types require a high pressure of the sphincter and pain in the epigastrium and/or right upper quadrant. Characteristics of SOD pain are as follows:

Episodes will generally last 30 minutes or longer.
Symptoms occur at different intervals.
Builds up to a steady level.
Severe to interrupt daily activities or require an emergency room visit.
Not relieved by a bowel movement, postural change, or antacids.
Exclusion of other structural disease that would explain the symptoms.
Pain may be present with nausea/vomiting, radiate to the back and shoulder, and may cause repeated night wakening.

Criteria for SOD Types 1, 2, and 3

SOD Type 1 patients will fulfill all of these three criteria:

Abnormal blood serum liver function test (LFT) focusing on two enzymes: ALT (Alanine aminotransferase, also known as SGPT- serum glutamic pyruvic transaminase) and; AST (Aspartate aminotransferase, also known as SGOT- serum glutamic oxaloacetic transaminase). Both enzyme levels need to be twice normal values on two different occurrences to be considered abnormal for SOD classification.

A dilated common bile duct (CBD) generally more than 12 mm on ultrasound or 10 mm on ERCP; a dilated CBD may also be determined through a CT scan or MRI.

Delayed drainage of contrast from the common bile duct after more than 45 minutes in the supine (horizontal) position during ERCP. The doctor injects contrast/dye into the ducts, so they are able to take images of the ducts and detect any narrowing, dilations or blockages. Images are taken by fluoroscopy, which is like a live x-ray video. If the dye takes longer than 45 minutes to empty, the patient has delayed drainage.

SOD Type 2 patients will fulfill one or two of Type 1 criteria.

SOD Type 3 patients present with high pressure (measured during ERCP) and pain syndrome only. None of the findings for SOD Type 1 are present.

	Biliary-type pain	Abnormal LFTs (a)	Dilated CBD (b)	Delayed drainage (c)
Type I	+	+	+	+
Type II	+	One or two of above		
Type III	+	None of the above		

(a) ALT and AST levels are more than two times normal values on at least two separate occasions.
(b) Common bile duct diameter greater than 12mm on ultrasonography, or greater than 10 mm on cholangiography.
(c) More than 45 minutes at ERCP while patient in supine position.

Criteria have been revised over the years to bump more patients into the SOD 3 category. At one time the biliary dilation requirement was only 8mm. Keep in mind this classification focuses on biliary-type SOD and is imperfect for describing all patients with biliary disorders. There is also the issue for patients having a functional pancreatic sphincter of Oddi disorder. In this case, Type 1 criteria are met, and the testing of pancreatic enzymes (amylase and lipase) will be abnormal. However, many patients, including me, had high pancreatic sphincter pressures upon manometry and pancreatic symptoms yet did not meet the SOD 1 criteria.

Although this is an imperfect way to determine SOD in every patient, I don't agree with the gastroenterologists who want to completely toss this classification system in the trash. There has been a large amount of discussion among gastroenterologists to do away with this classification system with no patient inclusion in the discussion. At some point, this section may become outdated for this reason. However, it is my hope the doctors still utilizing this system will continue to use it for the sake of SOD patients everywhere. We need a better diagnostic system, but throwing away the diagnosis as a whole is certainly not the answer and will ultimately gravely harm many patients.

Prevalence

According to the research article, "Sphincter of Oddi Dysfunction: Managing the patient with chronic biliary pain," the prevalence of SOD in the general population is 1.5%. SOD is seen in 1% of patients after cholecystectomy (gallbladder removal) but in 14%-23% of patients with the post-cholecystectomy syndrome (biliary pain with elevated liver enzymes). SOD can also be detected in 29% of patients with unexplained right upper quadrant pain and no evidence of gallstone disease, although due to symptom overlap many of these patients are not detected until after cholecystectomy. The prevalence of SOD in recurrent "idiopathic" (no cause can be found) pancreatitis ranges from 14.7%-72%.

SOD is more prevalent among middle-aged women for unclear reasons. A survey on functional gastrointestinal disorders confirmed that SOD affects females more frequently than males and indicated a high association with work absenteeism, disability, and healthcare use. Nowhere could I find research stating an exact or even presumed gender prevalence statistic for SOD. But, it is glaringly obvious if you visit any Internet SOD support group that over 90% of SOD patients are women.

I run one such group where there are two males out of 500 female members. Someone once told me that is because men generally don't join support groups. This is completely untrue. I belong to other health groups which have a 50/50 mix of men and women. Men have no problem participating in online support groups.

The Sphincter of Oddi Dysfunction Awareness and Education (SODAE) Network conducted two annual surveys, one in 2013 and the other in 2014. The results of which are on the website (http://www.sodae.org). 95-98% of respondents were female and the majority between age 30 and 50. Also, I have scoured through dozens of SOD studies on the National Institutes of Health's PubMed website. Anywhere from 75% to 92% of study participants were female. Hopefully, future research will discern gender prevalence and officially designate this a female-dominant disease like breast cancer.

Symptoms

The major presenting symptom in patients with SOD is abdominal pain as described previously. The pain is generally sharp, postprandial (after a meal), and located in the right upper quadrant or epigastrium, usually under the right ribcage, and may radiate to the back and up the shoulder. The pain may be associated with nausea and/or vomiting. Less common symptoms are fever, chills, jaundice, and bowel symptoms (constipation or diarrhea). SOD sufferers may also present with acute recurrent pancreatitis, which is extremely painful and almost always requires hospitalization.

The right side pain I had for many years was stabbing and quite severe. However, when my symptoms flared, it was nausea that took center stage. It was unrelenting--there from the minute I awoke in the morning till I closed my eyes at night. Still, that pain was what convinced a doctor and me that it could be SOD. It was a classic hallmark symptom.

It really is amazing that an area of the body smaller than the size of your pinky's fingernail could bring on such horrific pain radiating to such a broad area. Some women report SOD pain as being more painful than labor. Why is this? From a theoretical point of view, abnormalities of the sphincter of Oddi can give rise to pain by impeding the flow of bile and pancreatic juices resulting in ductal hypertension/pressure, ischemia (interruption of blood supply to a tissue or an organ) arising from spastic contractions, and "hypersensitivity" of the papilla. Although unproven, these mechanisms may act alone or together to explain the genesis of pain.

Another bothersome symptom is weight loss. It is not uncommon for SOD patients to lose significant amounts of weight unintentionally due to pain, nausea, vomiting, and/or malabsorption. Patients may become fearful of eating due to the possible onset of pain. As such, caloric intake becomes compromised. Nausea and vomiting can make food impossible to tolerate or keep down. Even if you want to eat and can tolerate food, SOD can alter bile and pancreatic enzyme output.

The body needs bile and pancreatic enzymes to metabolize and absorb nutrients. Too little of either means food is not properly broken down. This may cause food sensitivities and malabsorption. SOD can also cause an excess of bile and bile reflux into the stomach, which can impede absorption of nutrients. Too much bile in the stomach will neutralize stomach acid, which is vital to metabolizing and absorbing proteins, vitamins and minerals. Too much bile will also cause nausea, diarrhea, bacterial overgrowth, and absorption issues.

The majority of people I know would enjoy losing weight and actually voiced to me their envy of how thin I was. However, when you are already on the thin side and weight is flying off at lightning speed and severe weakness sets in, it is anything but desirable. It is frightening, to say the least.

Some patients have such a difficult time keeping weight on or the pain from eating is so severe, they have to get fed internally through a feeding tube or intravenously. I went from 135 pounds to 95 pounds in a nine-month period. I envied women with big butts because I completely lost mine. After that, I swore I would never again complain I needed to lose weight, though right now I weigh more than I ever have in my life. It is ok, though. I love having my body and health back. When I was thin and emaciated I was so weak I couldn't lift my child. Walking to the mailbox was exhausting.

While some SOD patients struggle with weight loss, others maintain their weight. Some gain weight. There really is no rhyme or reason when it comes to SOD. Some people may have severe SOD yet not lose weight because of other health conditions like thyroid disease, diabetes, or a hormonal imbalance. Others continue to eat poorly even if it causes pain and nausea. What I am saying is weight loss is not a definitive gauge of whether someone has SOD but fluctuations, especially significant weight loss, could be an indicator of SOD.

There may be debates on what constitutes SOD. Doctors and researchers will likely continue to change the diagnostic criteria, making it more inclusive than broad. It is quite possible a few rogue doctors will take it upon themselves to change the name of our diagnosis with little to no patient input. Even so, no one can argue with anatomy and physiology. This small muscular area is there, eligible for dysfunction and symptomology like any other body part, and will continue to be a hot topic for years to come.

Chapter 3: Causes of SOD

SOD is an elusive, difficult to diagnose disease that is even more difficult to treat. One reason for this is we don't know what causes SOD. Undoubtedly, if we knew the exact cause of SOD, we would likely have a solution for it. There may never be a cure, but knowing the cause could help find non-surgical treatments to put us in remission. For example, we know what causes most types of diabetes and, therefore, are able to control it with diet parameters, medications, and/or insulin replacement before it escalates into a stroke. Most digestive diseases are easily treated with medications or procedures. This is not the case for SOD.

Gastroenterology and Hepatology interviewed SOD specialist, Dr. Walter Hogan, for the article, "Diagnosis and Treatment of Sphincter of Oddi Dysfunction." When asked if there was a specific pathophysiologic cause that can be ascribed to sphincter of Oddi dysfunction, his response was as follows:

There is no specific cause and effect that has been determined with any scientific accuracy. The likelihood of getting a stricture or fibrosis from repetitive passage of stones or some inflammatory process is our standard explanation for what is termed sphincter of Oddi stenosis. Stenosis denotes a structural rather than a muscular defect. Causes of dysfunction are more speculative in terms of a neuromuscular component that is either abnormal or hyperactive and could conceivably increase pressure in the sphincter of Oddi and therefore cause intermittent flow obstruction. There is no verification of this explanation for these phenomena. They are best described clinically as functional disorders.

Some things are known about the sphincter of Oddi and should be explored in future research endeavors. Most notably, it has been documented that contraction and relaxation of the sphincter is regulated by neural and hormonal factors. Laboratory studies observing the effects of numerous peptides, hormones, and medications on the sphincter have suggested that there is a multifactor control mechanism of the sphincter of Oddi, and this mechanism affects the flow of bile.

In other words, the sphincter of Oddi controls the stop and go flow of bile, but also how continuous the flow occurs. Abnormalities in this control mechanism and/or process can result in SOD. Cholecystokinin (CCK), the hormone driving the gallbladder, and nitrates decrease the resistance offered by the sphincter.

In one study, biopsies of the sphincter of Oddi obtained at surgical sphincteroplasty (sphincters are sliced and sewn permanently open) from SOD patients, showed evidence of inflammation, muscular hypertrophy, fibrosis or adenomyosis within the sphincter of Oddi zone in approximately 60% of patients. In the remaining 40% with normal histology, a motor disorder was suggested. This is important for the purpose of proving SOD's existence.

Cholecystectomy (Gallbladder Removal)

The vast majority of SOD sufferers consistently reported their symptoms appeared or worsened after having their gallbladders removed. The term postcholecystectomy syndrome (PCS) describes the appearance of symptoms after cholecystectomy. According to the research site, Medscape, there are over 60 different etiologies of PCS. SOD is just one of those listed. It is ironic that a seemingly disposable organ could wreak such havoc once it is removed. Many people I know, including my brother, have had no issues or symptoms after their gallbladder was removed. In fact, most people feel better than ever. However, 10-15% of the population experience some form of PCS.

The 2014 SODAE Network patient survey asked when SOD symptoms began after gallbladder removal. The following are the results with the number of respondents and percentage out of 189 respondents:

Immediately: 27 (14%), Within first month: 47 (25%), One month-6 months: 24 (13%), 6 months-one year: 22 (12%), One year-5 years: 16 (8%), 5+ years: 15 (8%), Before gallbladder was removed: 23 (12%), Unsure or didn't have gallbladder removed: 15 (8%).

Clearly, SOD symptoms arose most frequently within the first six months following gallbladder removal.

No researcher or doctor, that I am aware, has been able to figure out why cholecystectomy seemingly gives birth to SOD. My SOD symptoms began a few weeks after my gallbladder was removed. The symptoms I had preceding my cholecystectomy were nothing like the symptoms I developed after the surgery. In fact, my gallbladder symptoms were mild in comparison to my SOD symptoms.

Though the American College of Physicians advises a conservative "wait and see" approach to gallbladder diseases, 600,000 are treated with cholecystectomies every year in the U.S. Cholecystecomy is not without risks. A study following 9,542 cholecystectomy patients over nine years found these risks: hemorrhage (224 cases, 2.3%), iatrogenic perforation of the gallbladder (1517 cases, 15.9%) and common bile duct (CBD) injuries (17 cases, 0.1%). Conversion to open operation was necessary in 184 patients (1.9%), usually due to obscure anatomy as a result of acute inflammation. The main postoperative complications were bile leakage (54 cases), hemorrhage (15 cases), sub-hepatic abscess (10 cases) and retained bile duct stones (11 cases). Ten deaths were recorded (0.1%).

I think removing 600,000 gallbladders a year is beyond excessive. Though I know many people with no PCS symptoms, I know much more with debilitating symptoms who wished they had never had their gallbladders removed. I am one of them. There are plenty of alternative treatments to gallstones or a low functioning gallbladder, which include:

<u>Endoscopic Retrograde Cholangiopancreatography (ERCP)</u>: a non-surgical procedure used to remove stones, sludge, treat SOD,

place stents or apply balloon dilatation to widen the bile duct, and use special x-rays for diagnostic purposes.

Extracorporeal Shock Wave Lithotripsy (ESWL): uses high-frequency sound waves to shatter cholesterol gallstones into pieces small enough to pass through the bile ducts into the intestines.

Ursodiol: a medication that suppresses cholesterol production in the liver, reducing the amount of cholesterol in bile, which can cause gallstones.

Natural Treatments: seek out a natural health practitioner to get your hormones in check naturally and prescribe supplements, herbs, dietary changes, and other natural treatments.

I was told my gallbladder was full of stones and looked diseased. Possibly then, I had no choice. But, I was never informed of alternatives to surgery or the justification there was an alternative to surgery. I can't tell you how many times someone has told me they didn't know why their gallbladder was removed. In fact, 9.5% of respondents of the 2014 SODAE Network survey said they did not know why their gallbladders were removed. Obviously, this is a huge problem.

I have a friend who had SOD symptoms. Her gallbladder was functioning fine and there was no sign of gallstones or gallbladder disease. Still, a surgeon convinced her to have her gallbladder removed on the chance it might make her feel better and resolve her mysterious symptoms. Well, it was no surprise to me. She did not feel better after the surgery or many months following the surgery. In time she recovered but I believe it was because she healed from whatever afflicted her in the first place, which was not her gallbladder. My question is how do these doctors and hospitals get the health insurance companies to approve removing an organ when there is zero sign of anything wrong with it or less invasive treatments could be trialed? How do they justify taking out someone's organ and provide no information about the possibility of SOD or PCS to the patient? I haven't met a single SOD patient who was told by their doctors that SOD or any PCS symptoms could arise from gallbladder surgery.

I am not advocating for anyone to not listen to their doctor. Just be informed. I would not have an organ removed ever again unless I knew it had to be removed—that my life depended on it. On the other hand, I know of a few SOD patients who actually benefitted from having their gallbladders removed. Their SOD symptoms improved after their cholecystectomy. These patients are definitely in the minority, but it needed to be mentioned.

I cannot begin to speculate on why a cholecystectomy would cause SOD. I personally think the hormone CCK plays a role. When I had a HIDA scan a few years ago, injection of CCK brought on instant SOD pain. Other SOD patients have reported this happening to them as well. Alternatively, I believe the digestive system becomes incredibly confused without one of its organs. Maybe some of us really need our gallbladders like we need other vital organs. There is a delicate synchronization of events that occurs during digestion.

In highly sensitive people, a subtle disruption in this process can produce significant consequences. An example of this is gastroparesis. Gastroparesis is a disorder where the stomach takes too long to empty. Even a slight alteration in gastric emptying time can result in disabling pain and nausea. Another example is how people recover after bariatric surgery. Most patients find the surgery to be successful. Most go on to lead healthier, happier lives. However, there are some who experience severe complications as their bodies have great difficulty adjusting to the new digestive process.

Hormones

One possible cause of SOD is hormones, especially knowing the majority of SOD sufferers are women. My SOD came to be after a cholecystectomy, which happened to be only a few years after having my second son. My SOD symptoms went nearly dormant during the pregnancy of my third son, a time when my female reproductive hormone levels surged. The symptoms returned with a vengeance after his birth, when these hormones plummeted. The same is true for many women I know with SOD. Nearly all report a reprieve from SOD symptoms during pregnancy and a resurgence after childbirth.

After my transduodenal sphincteroplasty, I still experienced some pain radiating on my right side, especially in the back to my right shoulder. It wasn't terrible but was there especially after eating. A few years after this I began experiencing unpleasant perimenopause symptoms. I allowed my gynecologist to prescribe a birth control pill that had a low dose of estrogen and progesterone with the hope it would level out my symptoms. The hormones not only improved my perimenopause symptoms, the pain radiating in my right side vanished entirely after a few months. Sadly, I had to go off the pills recently due to blood clot risks. Sure enough, the pain returned.

It makes sense SOD research would focus on hormones, right? Wrong. Though it is a female-dominant disease, research is sparse linking hormones to SOD. You would also think doctors would trial women on hormone therapy to treat SOD, right? Wrong. Very few are given this option. When I suggest exploring hormone therapy to female SOD patients, most complain about side effects they have experienced in the past from birth control. I can't imagine which is worse—birth control side effects or severe SOD side effects. One of the things I regret not trying prior to my ERCP and major surgery was hormone therapy.

It is important to talk about the hormonal differences in men and women and postulate which hormones could be at the center of SOD.

Hormonal Differences in Men and Women

The primary hormonal differences between men and women are the reproductive hormones, estrogens, and androgens (ex. testosterone). Estrogens have a profound effect on the gastrointestinal system, androgens not so much. Variations in these hormones not only affect the male and female reproductive system, but also the digestive system and digestive hormones. Men and women have the same hormones, yet there are variations in hormone levels and patterns, and there are differences in how the hormones interact with male and female bodies.

Estrogen/Progesterone

While estrogens are present in both men and women, they are usually present at significantly higher levels in women of reproductive age. The three major naturally occurring estrogens in women are estrone (E1), estradiol (E2), and estriol (E3). Probably the most obvious effect women's hormones have on the digestive system is estradiol's effect on the gallbladder. Women are twice as likely as men to have gallstones because estradiol raises cholesterol levels in the bile (the most common type of gallstone is the cholesterol gallstone) and slows gallbladder movement. One study on prairie dogs showed that sphincter of Oddi motility was significantly reduced during estrogen infusion. This meant that estrogen relaxed the sphincter.

Progesterone is another predominantly female hormone. The imbalances of estradiol and progesterone can influence the movement of food through the intestines—some by speeding the process up, causing diarrhea, nausea, and abdominal pain; and others by slowing things down and causing bloating and constipation.

In pregnancy, an increase in the hormone progesterone contributes to constipation by slowing the motility of intestinal contractions that move food down the digestive tract. In addition, progesterone causes the stomach's esophageal valve to relax, which could contribute to Gastroesophageal reflux disease (GERD). Since progesterone has a relaxation effect, maybe this is a reason SOD improves for most women during pregnancy, when progesterone levels are high. Progesterone also alters partitioning of hepatic bile between the gallbladder and small intestine and, therefore, gallbladder filling.

Relaxin

A woman with SOD once posted on the SODAE Network Facebook page how she thought the hormone relaxin was the reason her SOD subsided during her pregnancy. This got me thinking and wanting to learn more about this hormone. Relaxin is produced in both pregnant and nonpregnant females as well as in men. In women, relaxin rises to a peak within approximately 14 days of ovulation and then declines if ovulation does not lead to pregnancy. Relaxin levels rise and peak during the 14 weeks of the first trimester of pregnancy and then again at delivery. The role of relaxin in men is less clear. However, there is evidence that it may increase the movement of sperm cells in the semen.

Relaxin possesses an anti-inflammatory quality. It relaxes the pelvic ligaments, softens the pubic area, and increases cardiac output, renal blood flow, and arterial compliance. This could explain why SOD pain lessens during pregnancy. Relaxin may reduce ischemia (restriction in blood supply) and inflammation associated with SOD. For this reason, this woman's theory could be correct. Relaxin should be investigated for a possible connection with SOD, or at least as a treatment.

There are also several key hormones specific to the gastrointestinal system that could play a role in SOD. Although there are no glaring gender differences with these hormones, estrogen and progesterone affect some if not all. Therefore, the male/female difference is alive and well with these hormones too. The most common of these are cholecystokinin (CCK), secretin, and gastrin.

Cholecystokinin (CCK)

Cholecystokinin (CCK) is a peptide hormone that plays a key role in digestion and could very well be the key to unlocking the mysterious cause of SOD. CCK's role with the sphincter of Oddi is interesting. Ingestion of a fatty meal is followed by the release of cholecystokinin (CCK) which causes the gall bladder to contract and the sphincter of Oddi to relax. Coordination of gall bladder and sphincter of Oddi function may also be influenced by nerve bundles which connect the gall bladder and sphincter of Oddi via the cystic duct. Cholecystectomy may influence normal sphincter of Oddi function by disrupting this nerve pathway and altering its response to CCK.

After eating a meal, CCK is released into the bloodstream by endocrine cells located in the small intestine. Depending on which cells are receiving the CCK signal, the result can be either that digestive enzymes are delivered into the intestine from the pancreas, the gallbladder empties bile and food is shuttled faster through the intestine, or the person stops eating because they feel full. Cholecystokinin is also produced by neurons in the enteric nervous system and is widely and abundantly distributed in the brain. Studies also link CCK to panic attacks. This is interesting as most SOD sufferers report stress triggers their symptoms.

There really is no difference with CCK among men and women outside of the effect estrogen and progesterone have on it. Progesterone significantly affects gallbladder emptying in response to CCK by inducing a concentration-dependent relaxation of the gallbladder. In addition, it is well documented that estradiol regulates CCK and induces a relaxation of CCK-induced tension.

Other digestive hormones requiring attention are secretin and gastrin. Secretin functions as a type of fireman: it is released in response to acid in the small intestine, and stimulates the pancreas and bile ducts to release a bicarbonate base, which neutralizes the acid. All of this transiently increases the tone of the sphincter of Oddi.

Gastrin, found in the stomach, may play a role in SOD. Studies have shown stomach acid triggers the sphincter of Oddi to open and close properly. Most who suffer from SOD symptoms following cholecystectomy have higher serum levels of gastrin, likely caused by sphincter of Oddi hypomotility and duodenal-biliary reflux.

I could not find research studies on estrogen or progesterone affecting secretin or gastrin. That is not to say they don't have an effect. There just isn't any research on it. The same goes for around 30 other hormones, including those affecting the pituitary and adrenal glands which could have an effect on the sphincter of Oddi. Chandler Marrs, the founder of Hormones Matters (https://www.hormonesmatter.com/), has spearheaded fundraising campaigns in response to the lack of hormone research. Outside of her efforts, I am not aware of any other broad initiative to research how hormones affect us. I recommend visiting her website (https://www.hormonesmatter.com/) as she has been a supporter of SOD patients by publishing SOD articles and patient stories.

Though I have pointed out the hormonal differences in men and women and how female reproductive and other hormones affect the sphincter of Oddi, it is still unclear why statistically men rarely suffer from SOD. Possibly, it is the fluctuations themselves that make women more vulnerable and not the actual hormone level.

In other words, the sphincter of Oddi may favor a steady level of hormones throughout its lifespan. Women's hormone levels are far from consistent. We deal with variations every month throughout our cycle; and with pregnancy surges, the erratic fluctuations of perimenopause, and the near death of our hormones from menopause.

Furthermore, the sudden absence of a gallbladder may tip the scales over beyond what the sphincter of Oddi can handle. It certainly is a mystery that needs solving. We desperately need researchers to focus on this unchartered territory!

Prostaglandins

Our bodies experience pain through chemical messengers traveling through the body, and they end up passing these messages to the brain. Our brains then register this message as a 'pain' response and we feel that pain. This pain response alerts the body to a threat, example a cut, bodily trauma, inflammation within the body, etc. If you cut off these messengers, your brain will not register this pain. These chemical messengers are called prostaglandins and they are found throughout your body.

In general, prostaglandins act in a manner similar to that of hormones, by stimulating target cells into action. However, they differ from hormones in that they act locally, near their site of synthesis, and they are metabolized very rapidly. Their purpose is activation of the inflammatory responses at the sites of damaged tissue, and production of pain and fever. When tissues are damaged, white blood cells flood the site to try to minimize tissue destruction. Prostaglandins are produced as a result.

Prostaglandins are released by women during menstruation. For this reason, there may be a connection between why more women get SOD pain than men. In addition, they regulate smooth muscle activity (the sphincters are made up of smooth muscle) and glandular sections (the pancreas is a gland).

Medications, Alcohol, and Recreational Drugs

I am a proponent of taking as few medications as possible and when you do need medications, be aware of side effects. With the large number of side effects a drug can produce, SOD could be something that develops as an adverse reaction suddenly or over time. Simply put, we don't know how a person will react to any given medication.

Some medications are notorious for inducing sphincter of Oddi spasms. Morphine is at the top of the list. The majority of SOD sufferers will jump off a hospital gurney, screaming in pain if morphine is administered. In years past, morphine was actually used to diagnose SOD. The test was called the Nardi morphine-neostigmine provocation test.

Patients would be given doses of morphine and then the pain was rated before and after the test. At some point, the Nardi test was deemed unreliable by a few researchers and doctors and is no longer used by the majority of doctors as an indicator of SOD. In my opinion, this conclusion was not derived from anything evidence-based, but more from unreliable and unfounded opinions.

I can attest firsthand how painful the introduction of morphine was for my SOD. After my one and only ERCP and subsequent acute pancreatitis and sepsis, the doctors thought it was a great idea to give me morphine because I had trouble with oxymorphone (Dilaudid) during a previous hospital stay. Within seconds my sphincter was very angry and my SOD pain shot to an un-Godly number on the pain scale. I asked for meperidine (Demerol) but they wouldn't give it to me.

I've read in several research articles that Demerol is recommended for those with SOD pain over morphine or a synthetic morphine. The attending doctor told me they didn't even have Demerol and the only other pain relief option was Toradol, a NSAID. They tried giving me the Toradol but it barely touched the pain I was in. It was awful. My GI doctor came and advocated for me to get a fentanyl patch—anything to get me off the morphine drip. In my opinion, morphine absolutely can and should be used as an indicator for SOD. The morphine most definitely went straight to my sphincter area, causing my sphincter to scream in rage.

Strangely, I did not have this experience with other opioid medications—only morphine. Nearly every opioid pain medication has "spasm of sphincter of Oddi" as a side effect. Therefore, pain medication could be a double-edged sword and cause just as much pain as the original SOD pain. Another thing to consider is opioids could make nausea worse from the increased spasms. It is also a known contributor to gastroparesis and decreased intestinal motility which can cause pain, nausea, and bowel issues.

It is important the SOD patient find a pain medication that does not cause more pain in the long run. From my own experience conversing with other SOD patients, those who had the most difficulty achieving permanent, lasting pain or symptom relief were those who took opioid pain medications daily and for long periods.

An opioid medication you may not be aware even *is* an opioid medication is the anti-diarrhea medication, loperamide (Imodium). An SOD patient recently told me her spasms increased with hydrocodone, loperamide, and beef jerky. I completely forgot loperamide was an opioid until she mentioned it made her sphincter of Oddi spasm. This is why it stops diarrhea just as an opioid pain medication will constipate you. However, you can't get high from it because it does not cross the blood/brain barrier. If you have diarrhea, rather than reach for the loperamide, you may want to talk with your doctor about non-opioid alternatives.

Benzodiazepines (benzo) may cause SOD-like symptoms. I don't think it is the benzo itself that causes issues, but the interdose withdrawal and tolerance issues these drugs present. Many people with SOD end up on a benzo as it helps relax the sphincter and, as an added bonus, eases anxiety.

Interdose withdrawal is common with these drugs, meaning you could get relief from SOD symptoms with the benzo only to have terrible flares occur once it wears off. Also, you can quickly build up a tolerance to the benzo. I have met many people tapering off benzos or who quit the medication abruptly suddenly acquire SOD and pancreatic symptoms. Again, here is a situation where research is only minimally documenting this phenomenon but visit a few support groups and you will get a dose of reality.

Strangely, once these people went through withdrawal entirely, their symptoms improved or vanished. I hope researchers will study this class of drugs and the effect it may have on the sphincter and biliary and pancreatic systems, especially since so many SOD patients are on them. I will talk more about benzos in the chapter about medications.

I have not found research connecting alcohol and recreational drug usage with SOD. Alcohol, though, is reported as a common trigger of flares in many SOD patients. Most patients have to give up alcohol entirely as to avoid painful episodes. I would think most recreational drugs are bad for SOD just as they are bad for the body in general. The only recreational drug that may not be bad for SOD but, conversely, beneficial is marijuana, which I will also talk about in the medications chapter. I have never heard a single SOD patient complain that marijuana made their SOD worse, yet as with any medication or drug, you could be that one person in a thousand it does have an adverse effect upon.

Other Possible Causes

Less commonly, infections like Cytomegalovirus or Cryptosporidium, as may occur in AIDS patients, or a parasite like Strongyloides have caused SOD. Bacteria, viruses, and antibiotics all could affect the sphincter of Oddi. It was found that Sphincter of Oddi laxity (a relaxed sphincter) is associated with cholangitis (infected bile). It was proposed the cause was due to enhanced reflux of intestinal contents that changes the microenvironment. However, the microenvironment has not been investigated comprehensively.

It would be no surprise bacteria played a role in SOD. Our bacteria are like little engines, helping to control much of what occurs in our guts. My SOD flared after childbirth and an infection treated with antibiotics. Antibiotics disrupt the delicate balance of our microbiome.

Other possible causes are also those conditions mimicking SOD. See Chapter 12: If It is Not SOD What is It?

Chapter 4: Finding an SOD Doctor

Diagnosing SOD is generally not easy or straightforward. Since SOD can mimic other conditions, it often involves a complicated series of ruling out other diseases and conditions while subjecting the patient to many different tests. I wish it were as simple as going to the doctor, having blood drawn, getting an ultrasound, and waiting for a diagnosis. In this perfect scenario, the diagnosis would be definitive—undoubtedly either you had SOD or you did not. Unfortnately this is not the reality for most suffering from SOD. To say SOD is an elusive condition is an understatement.

Some of you may feel "intuitively" you have SOD. You have diligently combed the Internet and everything points to SOD as the cause of your woes. Alternatively, you may have been given an SOD diagnosis from a functional medicine practitioner or family physician and are satisfied with his or her conclusion. If either of these scenarios is true for you, and you want to stick to treatments of the natural kind or medications prescribed by your doctor you may not feel the need to obtain an "official" SOD diagnosis by an SOD specialist.

As long as you are able to function, have a decent quality of life, and your blood test results are normal, not having an SOD diagnosis may work for you. However, if you decide to go this route I encourage you to read this chapter to arm yourself with knowledge in case circumstances change. Of course, if your symptoms ever flare to the extreme--to the point you cannot eat or drink or pain is unbearable, an emergency room visit should be considered.

While in the emergency room, they will likely do initial bloodwork and an imaging study. At this time, it is imperative you are aware of the different imaging studies and their associated risks, which will be discussed in the next chapter. Some tests have minimal radiation or other risks while others have a potentially substantial risk.

The ease of diagnosing each SOD patient is never fluid. It is never a one size fits all process. One patient may have glaring symptoms and test results pointing to SOD. Other patients may have vague symptoms and perfectly normal test results, making diagnosis challenging. Traveling the road to an SOD diagnosis, or ruling out SOD, can be a long and winding journey, filled with wrong turns, speed bumps, and dead ends.

You will need an SOD GPS, in the form of this chapter and the next, to guide you along the way. The key is to follow these suggestions and never give up. Arm yourself with knowledge and a doctor who will take the entire journey with you. The most important thing you will need for diagnosing or ruling out SOD is a good SOD doctor.

Finding a qualified SOD doctor is the first and most important step in getting an accurate diagnosis. It is imperative that you only seek or rule out an SOD diagnosis from an "SOD doctor"—a doctor who will diagnose and treat SOD. The doctor you are looking for will likely be a gastroenterologist, depending on the country you live in. You can search online to find SOD doctor lists. As of this writing, The SODAE Network has an SOD doctor list on its website (http://www.sodae.org). If the list does not have a doctor close to you or for some reason the list and website become outdated, call around to gastroenterology groups in your area, preferably those affiliated with a major hospital.

Even if you find an SOD doctor on an online list, call and interview him or her or their staff. Ask if he or she tests for and treats SOD. Do not waste your time with a doctor who will not consider SOD as a diagnosis and most importantly, be aware some doctors do not believe the condition exists.

Make Sure the Doctor Diagnoses and Treats SOD

There are world-renowned medical institutions and clinics in the United States where patients are told SOD does not exist and their doctors will not consider it as a diagnosis. To lay claim that the biliary, pancreatic, and Oddi sphincters are the only parts of the human body 100% free from dysfunction or dysfunction of these sphincters could not cause debilitating symptoms is just plain impossible and irresponsible. No organ or body part is perfect and without the potential for defect and symptomology.

I cannot tell you how many times I have met someone in an online support group or forum who was given the run-around and wasted thousands of dollars traveling to a well-known medical establishment or clinic only to receive the wrong diagnosis because the doctors refused to acknowledge that SOD existed. One world-renowned clinic seems to churn out nothing but psychiatric diagnoses for women with SOD symptoms. Every woman I know who was ultimately diagnosed and treated for SOD who went to one of these clinic locations all left with a psychiatric diagnosis. This same clinic has treated men for SOD, but no women I have encountered.

There are many large hospitals and medical centers that still advertise information about SOD on their websites though they no longer acknowledge the condition. Most often, patients with SOD symptoms go to one of these hospitals under the impression they diagnose and treat SOD. They figure since it is a world-renowned clinic they will figure out the cause of their symptoms, including whether it could be SOD. These patients leave their appointments diagnosed with a minor digestive issue, a neuralgia, and/or a psychiatric condition. They report feeling blamed and shamed for their symptoms. Time goes by and their health continues to decline. Some give up their search for an SOD doctor, entrusting the doctors who told them SOD does not exist or they could not possibly have SOD.

After all, the medical center is well known, they must have all the answers, right? Wrong! Some of these patients lose their ability to work or raise their children, and end up with a poor quality of life. All of these things could have been avoided if they saw the right doctor from the beginning. Fortunately, some patients trust their instincts that something isn't right and that doctors are human and, as such, can make mistakes. They refuse to give up and eventually find an SOD doctor who is able to help them.

It isn't just big medical centers that refuse to acknowledge SOD, many small town doctors are of the same mindset. I was misdiagnosed with IBS for 13 years by my local doctors. It was manageable so I didn't have an issue with this diagnosis. However, when my symptoms became disabling, my local doctors not only refused to consider SOD as a diagnosis, they tried to tell my family and me that my problems were psychological in nature or that whatever I had would go away in time.

Carefully screen any doctor you intend to consult. If their office staff cannot give you a definitive answer as to whether the doctor is an "SOD doctor," do not book an appointment. I had pushy office staff book appointments for me only to find out later the doctor either knew nothing about SOD or did not believe in diagnosing it. My health declined rapidly in the course of a year, all because my local doctors wasted my time and did not believe in SOD.

Gastroenterologists are a dime a dozen where I live in upstate New York, but none who I saw were open to considering SOD as a diagnosis. A few who previously treated SOD stopped doing so around the same time I became ill. Others never heard of SOD and did not want to learn from me about it. Sadly, none of these doctors made an effort to refer me to someone who could rule out SOD. I did all of the legwork on my own to find an SOD doctor. This seems to be the case for most SOD patients.

Along my journey, I have met many other patients who clearly had all of the markers for SOD—abnormal liver enzymes, a dilated duct, and classic SOD symptoms. Though SOD was a strong possibility as the cause of these patients' symptoms, the doctors refused to consider it as a diagnosis or refer them to an SOD specialist. This peculiar disdain for acknowledging the existence of SOD is baffling. But more importantly, it is dangerous.

Do NOT waste your time with such doctors. Run! If they are not open-minded, any delay in obtaining an accurate diagnosis can be detrimental to your health. I have seen many patients subjected to questionable treatments though their condition was "unknown."

Some patients are diagnosed with a neuralgia and treated like lab rats. Their doctors perform nerve destroying treatments that are not evidence-based. In a few cases, nerve treatments helped the pain for a period of time. However, treating nerve pain does nothing for other SOD symptoms like nausea, vomiting, weight loss, or bowel issues.

Some who read this guide may not have SOD. They may go through all of the SOD tests only to discover they do not have it. What is important is that each and every one of us receives an accurate diagnosis. It is highly likely that if you go through the extensive battery of tests for SOD, you will find your way to a diagnosis that explains your symptoms and will determine appropriate treatment.

If you find an SOD doctor—one who believes in SOD and is knowledgeable about the condition you will also want a doctor who is compassionate, open-minded, smart, fair, honest, respectful and spends quality time with you. It is kind of like dating. If only there was an online dating service for patients and SOD doctors, life would be so much easier.

I know it is near impossible to pinpoint a doctor's qualities before meeting him or her. In my experience, the best way to find out about a doctor is from other patients. Look for online reviews. There are websites where patients can rate their doctor. Some include patient comments. Plug the term "doctor rating" into any search engine and the top doctor rating sites will appear. Some I have used are www.vitals.com, www.healthgrades.com, www.zocdoc.com, and www.ratemds.com. I personally will not see a doctor who has less than a four-star rating on these sites. My health is a life or death matter. I take it very seriously and refuse to have substandard doctors on my care team.

Another way to learn about a doctor is through online support groups and forums. This is how I found the SOD doctor who diagnosed me. I had to travel halfway across the United States but it was worth it. Rarely have I seen a patient dissatisfied after seeing an SOD doctor recommended by another patient. The only instance I have witnessed this was when a doctor suddenly did an about face and no longer believed in or treated SOD. This is a reason why you should still ask the office staff of a recommended doctor whether he or she diagnoses and treats SOD before scheduling an appointment.

I cannot impress upon you enough that finding the right SOD doctor is the most important thing you can do. You are already sick. Trust me, if you go to a doctor or several doctors who mistreat you, refuse to validate your symptoms, and who are not open minded to SOD it will make you sicker from the traumatization and prolongation of symptoms.

Reality: You May Need to Travel

If your health insurance will pay for an out of state doctor, and you either have or can raise enough money to travel, I strongly encourage you to travel to see a top notch SOD doctor. As I mentioned, I had to do this and wished I had done it from the beginning, avoiding the nightmare I went through with local doctors. If you ask the doctor's staff, they will likely be able to recommend a hotel that offers a medical discount. My mother and I stayed in a very nice hotel at a great "medical" rate within walking distance to the doctor's office and hospital.

Air travel is expensive but you can search online for good fares. Let the SOD doctor's staff know you want to try a few different dates and ask if they could give you a few appointment options to allow you to find the best travel deals. If you go to a discount travel site, be sure to use the tool where you can search two to three days before and after your desired day of travel. This is an important tool to find the best rate.

Also, some major metropolitan cities have a few airports to choose from, so be sure to also check off the box to search nearby airports. If you are not airline savvy, ask friends and family if they know how to reserve flights online and to help find you the best rates.

There is usually someone we know who is familiar with travel sites. Of course, you could also contact a travel agency to help you find a good rate.

Whatever you do make sure you pay extra for a refundable fare or travel insurance. This way if you are too ill to travel you won't lose out on the fare. Some airlines will give you a full credit to be used for a future flight or a refund. Others, unless you have trip insurance, will not reimburse you anything or will only give you a partial credit.

Another option is to find an SOD doctor within driving distance who takes your insurance. I know many SOD patients who drive several hours to see a good SOD doctor. Often they have to cross state lines. The only financial issue, besides gas, that may arise is if you need a procedure that will land you in the hospital for a day or more. You may not need a hotel room, but your loved one(s) may. Distant relatives and friends can come in handy in these situations for a place to crash.

Many health insurance policies, unfortunately, are restrictive about which doctors you can see. I have had policies that allowed me to see nearly any doctor, anywhere in the United States. Then, there was the year when my husband's health insurance changed and I could only see doctors in my area. It was awful. No local doctor acknowledged or understood SOD, so as you can imagine it was a bleak year.

If this is the case for you, your health insurance policy may allow you to go out of network if there is absolutely no doctor to serve your needs. It is difficult to prove this. If it looks like your health insurance plan won't be changing anytime soon, at least find a local doctor open minded to SOD who, if unable to diagnose you, will advocate on your behalf to the insurance company to justify out of network treatment. I honestly couldn't find such a doctor but that doesn't mean you can't.

I know patients with SOD who won this argument after they found a doctor to advocate for them. If you are in a country where health insurance isn't an issue like it is in the U.S., congratulations! That being said, I do know, from the people I have met online, there is an SOD doctor shortage in most countries. This is beyond frustrating and will hopefully change.

The First Appointment

Many specialists, especially sought-after SOD doctors, are booked months in advanced. It took me one to two months to get an appointment with local gastroenterologists and three months for the out of town world-renowned SOD gastroenterologist. It was frightening to wait three months for an appointment as I was drastically losing weight, experiencing muscle atrophy, and living with constant nausea and pain. It may as well have been a year. That three months felt like forever.

Over time, I figured out a way to get an appointment sooner. First, when I needed an appointment sooner, I asked to be placed on a cancellation list. Therefore, I would be called when a cancellation came in, depending on where I ranked on the list. Sounded easy, but I often waited and waited and waited for that call. I was perplexed. Why weren't they calling me? People cancel all the time. I have canceled many appointments in my lifetime.

One day I was complaining about this to a friend of mine who worked for a large doctor's practice. She told me the cancellation list was only as good as the person holding the list. She informed me that some office workers were religious about ensuring cancelled appointments get filled by those on the list and on a first come basis. Other workers completely neglected to reach for the list to make these phone calls. Instead, they filled cancellations with whoever called next asking for an appointment.

A few days after making your appointment, start calling several times a week asking if there are any cancellations or openings. My most successful days securing appointments were Friday afternoon and Monday mid-morning. I think in some cases the office staff got so sick of my repeated calls they invented an appointment slot for me! Today, I never wait for more than a month for an appointment. Heck, if I called every day instead of several times a week I probably would have secured an appointment in a week or two. That old saying, "the squeaky wheel gets the grease," rings true.

Be prepared at the first appointment. Treat this appointment as if you were interviewing someone for a job or someone to care for your child. Prior to the appointment write down your questions. This doesn't mean you immediately slam the poor doctor with a million questions. Allow the doctor to physically examine you and ask you questions first. The doctor will ask why you are seeing him/her and what symptoms you are experiencing. Whatever you do, do not walk into your first doctor's appointment telling the doctor you have SOD or rattle off everything you learned about SOD from this book or online. It is the doctor's job to diagnose you, not for you to diagnose yourself. By all means, do let the doctor know you suspect SOD as a possible diagnosis, but leave the rest in his or her hands.

Tell the doctor when the symptoms started. Often SOD-like symptoms start after the patient's gallbladder was removed. If this is not the case for you, try to remember any significant events that led up to the symptoms. Did you have a child? Did you start a new medication or go off an existing medication? Were you under a lot of stress? Be sure to mention any symptoms you have and any you had before this all started.

Even if you had symptoms in the beginning that have since subsided, let him or her know. Describe the location and intensity of your pain as best you can. Is it stabbing or dull? Is it only under the rib or does it spread to the sides or back? Does it shoot up your shoulder? Have you noticed a trigger for the pain, i.e. a specific food, beverage, activity, or that time of the month for women? Tell the doctor your most troublesome symptom. Maybe it isn't pain but is constant nausea. Tell the doctor which tests you have already had and which doctors you have seen. Do not rely solely on the intake form you may have completed. Some doctors or their staff do not read them fully.

After the physical exam, ask your questions. Ask which tests he or she will perform and in what order. Ask what the doctor will do if all standard tests are fairly normal. What will be the next step? And the next step after that? Is this doctor open to performing an endoscopic ultrasound or ERCP with manometry (defined in the next chapter) to test pressure? Or, will he or she forego these tests and go straight to treatment options, basing the diagnosis on less invasive studies?

Some doctors may not like to discuss every possible test and rather focus on one test result at a time. What is important, though, is for the patient to know that the doctor is committed to exhausting any and all possibilities, within patient safety, to pinpoint the cause of the symptoms.

If your doctor seems amenable, ask him to describe an estimated timeline of if this test is normal, then such and such will be the next test and the next, and so on, and the timeframe of each process. If my local doctors had been more transparent about the diagnosis and treatment process, my anxiety would have been less, symptoms a little better, and life a bit easier. The unknown is not a good place for a patient who is suffering. Arming the patient with as much information as possible and practicing full disclosure is best practice. Ask if there are any other possible diagnoses for the symptoms you have. If indeed you have SOD, what are the treatments this doctor prefers to use?

Assuming you have found a good SOD doctor, the next chapter focuses on which tests are used to diagnose SOD.

Chapter 5: Diagnostic Tests

You have an SOD doctor and now the real fun begins. Hopefully, you will only need one or a few of the tests listed in this chapter. Regardless, it is important to know about all of the SOD tests even if you never end up having them. Knowing the risks involved with some scans and procedural tests may save your life in the long run. More is not always better in the world of diagnostic testing.

Which tests your doctor orders may ultimately depend on how severe your symptoms are. For example, if your symptoms can be managed with medication, the point of having a risky test is not justified. However, if your symptoms persist though many treatments have been trialed, and each test is coming up normal or only slightly abnormal, this chapter will help you decide whether to follow through with more extensive, risky testing.

Bloodwork

Bloodwork should always be ordered. A comprehensive metabolic profile is standard. It will show the status of your liver, kidneys, and electrolytes. Ask the doctor to include an order to measure your pancreatic enzyme levels as elevated levels could indicate a problem with the sphincters and ducts. If you have lost weight rapidly you may be malabsorbing nutrients and need your vitamin and mineral levels checked.

Inflammation and autoimmune disease markers may also be measured. No blood test result will definitively show you have SOD. Elevated liver enzymes could be any disease affecting the liver or bile duct. The same goes for pancreatic enzymes. If you search online for information on these common tests, you will find an endless list of possible diseases and conditions coinciding with test indicators. Therefore, bloodwork is just a complementary indicator of SOD. It is a starting point.

Many with SOD have normal, often perfect, bloodwork. Keep in mind, bloodwork does not always show what is really going on. Some end stage liver cirrhosis patients have perfectly normal liver enzyme levels. More unsettling is the majority of people with pancreatic cancer have perfect bloodwork and scans until tumors develop. Before my transduodenal sphincteroplasty, I weighed 95 pounds (40 pounds under my normal weight). I had significant muscle wasting. I was barely able to function due to severe dizziness bordering on fainting much of the time. I was so weak that walking from the car into a doctor's office wore me out. I had to use a wheelchair if I had to get from one end of a hospital to another. The chronic pain and nausea were debilitating.

Although my blood pressure was very low, my bloodwork and scans were perfectly normal. It made no sense. There are literally hundreds, possibly thousands, of diseases that cannot be detected through routine bloodwork and scans. Only very specialized tests can detect some conditions. SOD is no different.

Another concern is the interpretation of the results. Too often doctors may report that a result is normal even though it is just shy of abnormal. It is a good idea to obtain copies of all bloodwork, scans, and procedural results for this very reason.

I was fainting and white as a ghost at one point after my surgery. I saw my ferritin level was dangerously low, an indication I was anemic. My total iron was just shy of being abnormally low. For whatever reason, my doctors did not take it seriously. I had to advocate persistently for iron infusions. Eventually, I had a few iron infusions. Color returned to my face and I felt much better. Another time my bloodwork showed I was borderline dehydrated. I came close to blacking out a few times.

My doctor didn't think it was a problem because my bloodwork was still within the normal range. I had to go to the emergency room and get fluids and electrolytes a number of times which helped me feel better and the dizziness resolved. I learned to advocate for fluids and electrolytes. Remember that bumper sticker,

"Question Authority?" Practice that but in a diplomatic, empowered manner.

One of the best things I did was go to a naturopath. He ordered a series of alternative tests—most of which were costly and not covered by my insurance. I had a comprehensive stool analysis, organic acids/metabolic analysis test, and saliva hormone profile. The stool analysis showed, not surprisingly, that I had a shortage of pancreatic enzymes.

Also, my "good" gut bacteria were low. The organic acids/metabolic analysis test used urine and blood to measure malabsorption and dysbiosis; cellular energy and mitochondrial metabolism; neurotransmitter metabolism; vitamin deficiencies; and toxin exposure and detoxification need. The results of these tests were consistent with some of my symptoms. The saliva hormone test showed my cortisol was all whacky--too high in the morning and in the evening. My adrenals were in overdrive and fatigued. My progesterone and estrogen were super low, which was no surprise as I suspected low hormones contributed to my SOD.

Conventional doctors rarely acknowledge the efficacy of these tests though there is evidence to the contrary in medical journals. Regardless, I recommend exploring them particularly to measure nutritional status.

Review Your Imaging Reports and Bloodwork

Review your imaging reports as well as your bloodwork. I was told my bile duct was "normal" the entire time I was at my sickest. I was diagnosed with the controversial SOD Type 3 because I didn't meet the criteria for Type 1 and 2. I remembered a few doctors telling me my duct was mildly dilated. I grew curious, wondering if by chance I was misdiagnosed and actually had SOD Type 2. After reviewing my imaging reports, I discovered my duct was consistently three to four times its normal size. During my worst SOD days, my biliary duct ranged from 9mm to 11mm. Medical sources are inconsistent on what is considered "dilated."

For the SOD typing classification, the bile duct is presumed to be dilated if it is greater than 12mm on ultrasonography or 10mm on ERCP. I was 1mm off. However, it is important I mention I am a small-framed woman. I read once that most reference ranges, be it imaging, bloodwork, and pharmaceutical testing, are based on a 200-pound man and that the average diameter of the bile duct is 4.1mm. According to the article, "Sphincter of Oddi Dysfunction and Pancreatitis," the upper limit of normal (highest normal) for common bile duct diameter is 7 mm, a cut off of 10 mm or 12 mm potentially leaves a large number of patients misdiagnosed.

Long since I had the sphincteroplasty, my bile duct has been normal, consistently 3mm and under on imaging studies for three and a half years now. Turns out I have a tinier duct than the average person. Therefore, when it was dilated, it may have seemed "slightly dilated" but for my anatomy, it was indeed prominently dilated. Now, when people ask which type of SOD I had, my answer is, "Type 2."

I am by no means telling you to get a copy of an actual scan and try and interpret it. This is pretty much impossible for a lay person. Do not even attempt to interpret the visual of an ultrasound or CT scan. You will be wasting your time. This is why radiologists are medical doctors and go to school for a dozen years. Instead, request copies of the imaging report and read the report in its entirety. You can also try to get a second opinion regarding the results. Request this from your GI doctor or primary care doctor.

Recently, trying to make sense of my pancreatic attacks, I requested a copy of my MRCP/MRI report. The doctor who ordered the study told me everything was normal—his exact words. I read the report and it said I had what they presumed was pneumobilia, i.e. air at the entrance of the ducts. A research paper from the *Journal of Emergency Medicine* stated pneumobilia, or air within the biliary tree of the liver, suggests an abnormal communication between the biliary tract and the intestines, or infection by gas-forming bacteria. It went on to say that one of most common conditions associated with pneumobilia included an incompetent sphincter of Oddi.

My new GI doctor was concerned about the amount of gas in my intestines upon physical examination so he "prescribed" activated charcoal, which mops up gas. I was hesitant but when I saw the report, I started taking it. Within a few days, the attacks and pain lessened when I'd take the charcoal.

I also had scarring in my pancreatic duct show up on my earlier endoscopic ultrasound reports. Everything else looked ok but obviously something was wrong. I was told my test results were perfectly normal. I beg to differ. There is a story behind every scar on our body. Why would it not be different with scarring on a duct? I am not a doctor but believe even minor findings should be taken seriously and discussed with the patient. So, again, "normal" isn't always normal. This is why I like the growing field of functional and naturopathic medicine where practitioners look at the whole picture and consider results in diagnosing disease and tailoring treatments even if the results are within "normal" parameters.

Imaging Studies

Imaging studies can offer a good visualization of your digestive system. Most, however, cannot measure how well your system is functioning. Since SOD is a functional disorder, the main reason your doctor will order an imaging study is to rule out other conditions which may be causing your symptoms. In addition, he or she will want to know if your bile and/or pancreatic duct are dilated as this is one of the hallmark signs of SOD. Keep in mind, though, that a dilated bile and/or pancreatic duct does not guarantee you have SOD. There are numerous other conditions which cause dilated ducts.
and other structures within your body. If you are a woman who has been pregnant, you have most likely experienced an ultrasound to track the growth and health of your baby. Ultrasound can show biliary or pancreatic duct stones and ductal changes. It can measure the size of the liver, pancreas, and ducts as well as show tumors and cysts.

An external ultrasound does not produce a good snapshot of the

pancreas as it sits behind the stomach, and is not a good tool for showing other organs, blood vessels, or tissue in great detail. If your ultrasound is normal or your doctor or the radiologist finds something needing a better visual, he or she will likely order a CT scan or MRI as the next step. Most insurance companies
Imaging studies vary. Some use radiation. Some don't. Some are invasive but most are non-invasive.

You have likely had an x-ray or know of someone who has had an x-ray. The X-ray is an example of an imaging study that is an easy, quick way to take a snapshot of your insides. Although an x-ray is useful for detecting broken bones, or possibly a large tumor or mass, gallstones, or show if you are constipated, it does not produce a detailed snapshot of the organs or the ducts. For this reason, your SOD doctor will likely order an ultrasound as the first imaging study.

Ultrasound

Ultrasound is an imaging method that uses high-frequency sound waves to produce images of the inner workings of your organs require a series of tests before they will approve payment for costlier or invasive imaging studies.

CT Scan

A CT (Computed Tomography) scan combines x-ray with computerized technology to produce highly detailed images of organs, blood vessels, and tissues. Sometimes an iodine or barium based contrast agent, also known as a dye, will be administered either orally, rectally or via injection. The contrast will produce an enhanced visual of specific organs, blood vessels, and/or tissues. Some people, especially those with kidney disease, cannot tolerate the contrast agent.

Although contrast is often preferred, it isn't necessarily needed to capture a visual. CT scans are rather quick and easy with few restrictions, unlike MRI. That being said, CT scans carry the most radiation risk of all imaging methods. According to Consumer Reports, "CT scans emit a powerful dose of radiation, in some cases equivalent to about 200 chest X-rays, or the amount most people would be exposed to from natural sources over seven years."

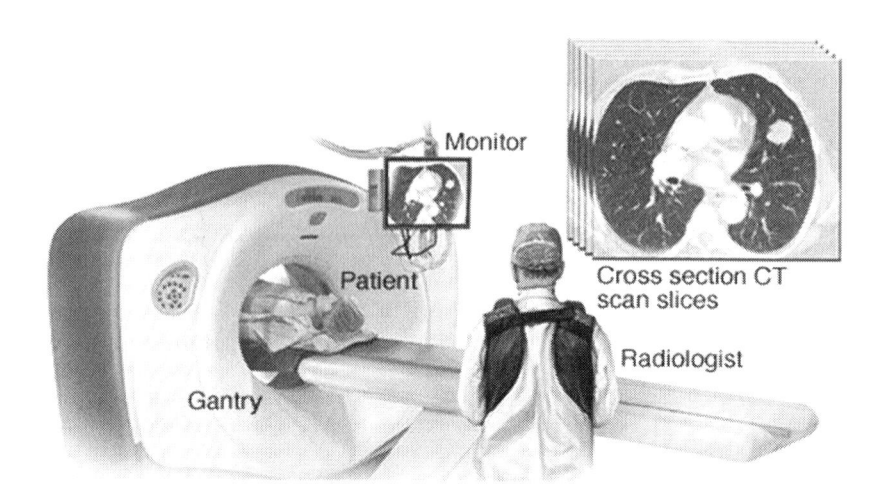

Every time I landed in an emergency room the ER doctor would order a CT scan. I didn't see this as a problem in the beginning of my journey but am now very concerned about the amount of radiation exposure I have endured throughout my illness. I have had over a dozen CT scans. Most were not necessary. I did not know any better.

Today, if I am in the ER or hospital, I refuse CT scans unless it is a life or death situation. I say this not to scare you but to inform you. A CT scan in the beginning of the SOD diagnostic journey is pretty much standard and could reveal a glaring condition that needs to be addressed. Beyond that, I'd ask if there is an alternative imaging study the doctor can recommend.

MRI/MRCP

MRI (Magnetic Resonance Imaging) uses strong magnets and radio waves instead of radiation to create images of the digestive organs. It is not as detailed as a CT scan but is more detailed than an ultrasound. Some people who have implantable devices cannot get an MRI, and you must remain absolutely motionless for long periods of time. SOD doctors will likely order an MRCP (magnetic resonance cholangiopancreatography) rather than an MRI.

An MRCP is basically the same thing as an MRI, but it specifically evaluates the liver, gallbladder, bile duct, pancreas, and pancreatic duct for disease. Often a contrast called gadolinium is used. It is a rare earth mineral and is less likely to cause an allergic reaction compared to the iodinated contrast agents used in CT scanning. I never had a problem with it but did know a woman with Lyme disease who had difficulty detoxifying heavy metals and was sick with weird symptoms for a few months after receiving gadolinium.

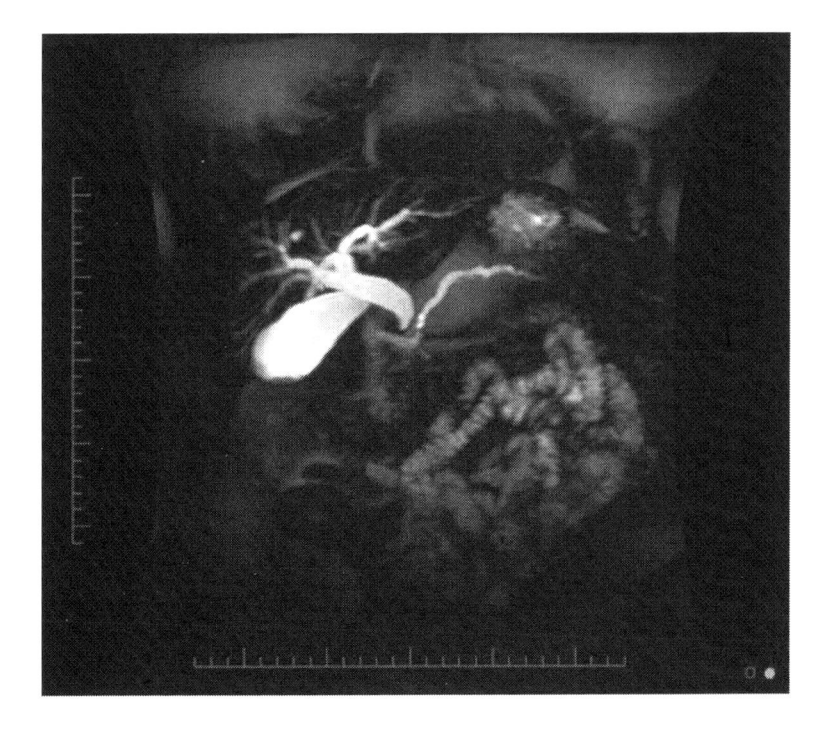

HIDA Scan (Cholescintigraphy)

A HIDA scan is a test done by nuclear medicine physicians to diagnose bile duct obstructions, gallbladder disease, bile leaks, and signs of SOD. After cholecystectomy, SOD may show on a HIDA scan as a partial common bile duct obstruction. You will likely be placed on your back for the test as it can take an hour or more. A radioactive tracer will be injected into a vein in your arm. The tracer travels through your bloodstream to your liver and is then excreted by the bile-producing cells. The radioactive tracer travels with the bile from your liver into your gallbladder and through your bile ducts to your small intestine.

Emptying delayed by more than two hours or a prolonged half-time can help identify the sphincter of Oddi as a potential cause for your symptoms. However, it cannot differentiate between other conditions such as stenosis and dyskinesia. Pretreatment of CCK hormone may improve the sensitivity for its detection. CCK is used to induce gallbladder contractions and is generally used to measure gallbladder functioning. A HIDA scan, however, lacks the adequate resolution to identify dilation and stricture. It also does not provide imaging of the pancreas, pancreatic duct, or functioning of the pancreatic sphincter.

Endoscopy and Colonoscopy

Endoscopy literally means "looking inside." A scope is put through the mouth, down the throat, into your esophagus, stomach, and duodenum until it reaches the entrance to the pancreatic and biliary ducts. This scope can take images and retrieve biopsy samples of tissue of the esophagus, stomach, and duodenum. Many upper gastrointestinal conditions like ulcers, celiac disease, bacterial infections, bile gastritis, hiatal hernia, and some cancers can be diagnosed via an endoscopy.

However, an endoscopy in no way can definitively diagnose SOD. This procedure is used to rule out other conditions which could be causing your symptoms. An endoscopy procedure carries few complications. Most complications are related to the anesthesia. If you have any loose teeth, the tube could inadvertently force a tooth to come out. The tube can also irritate the throat and esophagus for several days.

A colonoscopy is an endoscopic evaluation of the large intestine or colon. Lower gastrointestinal issues like diverticulitis, polyps, Crohn's disease, ulcerative colitis, hemorrhoids, and some cancers can be diagnosed through colonoscopy. Like an endoscopy, a colonoscopy will not diagnose SOD. It is used to rule out other possible causes of your symptoms. Patients often say the worst part of the colonoscopy is the prep the day before the procedure in which they have to ingest a good amount of a laxative solution and as such spend much of their day and evening in the bathroom. There are few risks. Like with an endoscopy, patients sometimes react to anesthesia. Other than that a rare complication is bowel perforation.

For both the endoscopy and colonoscopy, you will not be able to eat or drink after a certain time of the day or evening before the procedure. These are considered outpatient procedures, meaning you will be at the hospital or endoscopy center for part of a day and rarely need to be admitted overnight. Due to the sedation used during the procedure, you will not be able to drive for 24 hours. Most people do not remember their endoscopy or colonoscopy due to the sedation involved.

Endoscopic Ultrasound (EUS)

EUS is essentially an endoscopy scope with an ultrasound attachment on the end. The prep and after-care is the same as an endoscopy. EUS can be used to diagnose diseases of the pancreas, bile duct, and gallbladder when other tests are inconclusive or conflicting. In respect to SOD, an EUS cannot measure sphincter function. It can however, identify ductal changes like strictures and dilated ducts that could be caused by SOD.

Since many people with SOD also have issues with their pancreas,

EUS is a good visual option in comparison to ERCP, which can cause acute pancreatitis. Another advantage of the EUS is a needle can be used to obtain a biopsy of the pancreas tissue to detect cellular abnormalities.

EUS is also used to evaluate known abnormalities, including lumps or lesions, which were detected at a prior endoscopy or were seen on x-ray tests, such as a CT scan. EUS provides a detailed image of the lump or lesion, which can help your doctor determine its origin and help treatment decisions.

Endoscopic Retrograde Cholangiopancreatogram (ERCP)

ERCP is similar to an endoscopy and EUS as it uses a scope and prep and aftercare is similar. With an ERCP, a catheter is attached to the end of the scope. This catheter can inject a dye into the biliary and pancreatic ducts which will help to produce high-quality x-rays of the ducts and organs. Other catheters and guidewires may be used to enter the ducts or measure the sphincter and ductal pressures (manometry). ERCP with sphincter of Oddi manometry is considered the "gold standard" in the diagnosis of SOD.

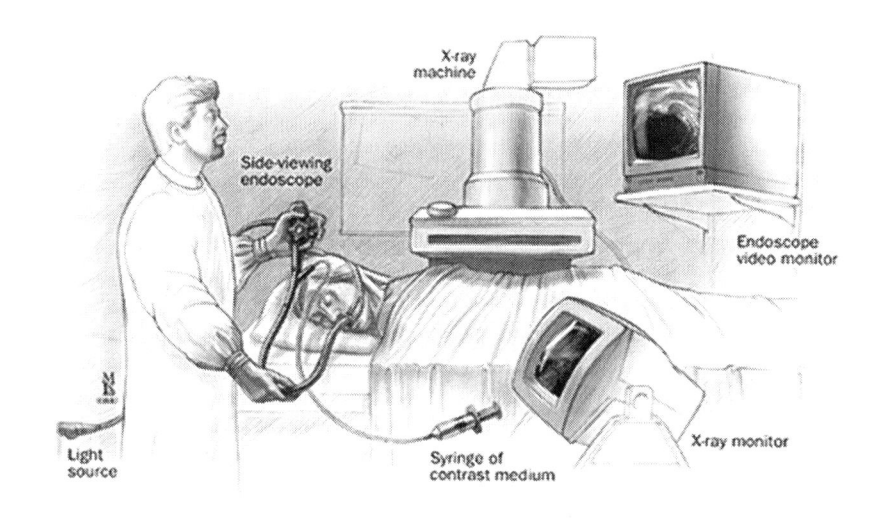

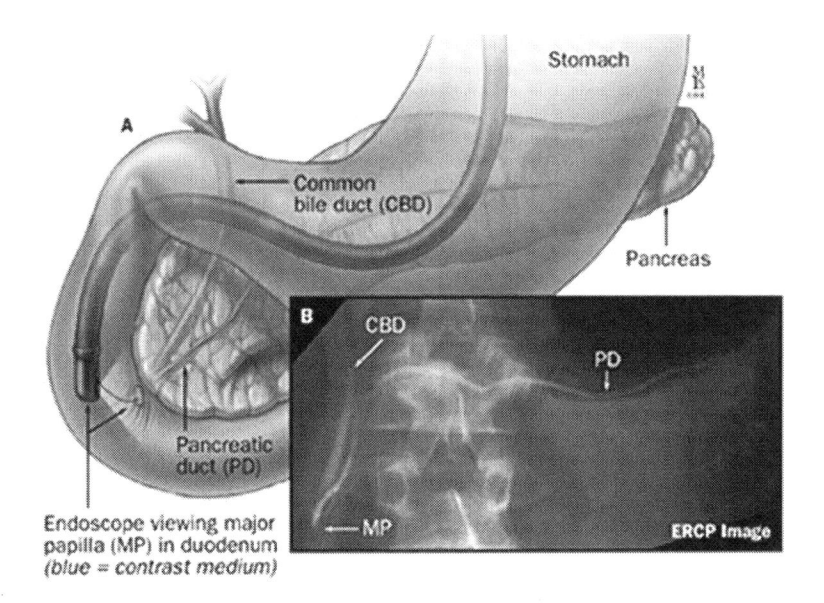

Figure labels: Stomach; Common bile duct (CBD); Pancreas; Pancreatic duct (PD); Endoscope viewing major papilla (MP) in duodenum (blue = contrast medium); B — CBD, PD, MP, ERCP Image

Diagnostic and Therapeutic Endoscopy defined sphincter hypertension as basal sphincter pressures above 40 mmHg and is considered manometric evidence of SOD. Theoretically, elevated sphincter pressures indicate the sphincter is prone to spasm, causing SOD symptoms. The higher the manometric reading, the worse the sphincter spasms. Though it is the gold standard, even ERCP with manometry is not foolproof. Because of inconsistent results, manometry has become as controversial as SOD itself. One problem I found in researching manometry information is that it is not as standardized as it was a few decades ago.

This means that doctors have moved away from this method of diagnosing SOD; and there is no reliable data collection system gathering information on manometry results, symptoms, treatments, and outcomes. Subsequently, there is a lack of data sharing. Though studies show manometry does not contribute to acute pancreatitis, SOD doctors will perform a sphincterotomy, cutting the sphincter during ERCP, yet not bother to conduct manometry.

Many factors could affect manometry results. For example, patients sometimes incorrectly report medications they ingested the day prior to the ERCP. Even if a patient is told to not take medication within 12 hours of the procedure, the drug may still be in their systems due to the individual's metabolism and its effect on a drug's metabolism and excretion. Aside from anticholinergics, nitrates, calcium channel blockers, glucagon, opioids, and cholinergic agents, we don't know the extent of effect most drugs have on the sphincter.

In fact, it is not known for certain the hypertensive relationship of benzodiazepines or propofol, the primary anesthetics used during an ERCP, on the sphincter. Fentanyl is often used during an ERCP. Fentanyl is an opioid, which can cause the sphincter to spasm. Another issue, which I discussed earlier, is the anatomical differences in people, i.e. 200 lb. man vs. 100 lb. woman. Could these differences affect manometric readings? Probably not, but it is worth mentioning.

As you can see, reaching a definitive diagnosis of SOD is challenging, if not impossible, using traditional methods. Some patients have normal findings and only after an invasive intervention successfully relieves the patient's symptoms is it obvious the patient actually had SOD. We obviously need more research into finding the true cause(s) of SOD. I know; I must sound like a broken record about research, but it will enable us to identify the best way of diagnosing SOD.

Chapter 6: Natural Treatments

Throughout much of my SOD experience, some of the most beneficial "remedies" were of the holistic and natural kind. Simple remedies like deep breathing, meditation, yoga, and dietary changes helped me to manage my severe SOD pain from 1998 till 2011. It took nearly a year after the onset of symptoms to nail down which things helped and a few months after that for all of these natural treatments to get me back to a normal life. But it *did* happen.

Sadly, during the years 2011-2012 when my SOD symptoms were disabling, my tried and true natural treatments ceased to help. I tried some of the other treatments listed in this chapter but unfortunately, my symptoms proved to be impenetrable. I quickly gave up on natural treatments. Today I look back and wish I had not given up so quickly and instead continued to try natural treatments till one helped.

One of the reasons I stopped seeking natural treatments was cost. During that period, I constantly feared I would become disabled, which did end up happening. I worried about money and needed a cure fast. I resorted to only seeking care from medical doctors or practitioners who accepted my health insurance. Unfortunately, I still ended up doling out thousands of dollars in copays with few positive results. I would get frustrated when friends suggested I see a natural health practitioner. Didn't they know I didn't have hundreds of dollars to shell out? Also, my symptoms were quite severe so there was an extreme sense of urgency I had that I thought only traditional allopathic medical doctors could fix.

It wasn't that traditional doctors were all that cheaper than natural practitioners. In fact, in the end, I spent much more on traditional doctors. However, it was easier to justify spending a $25.00 copay here, a $40.00 copay there. In time, though, those little copays added up after going to multiple specialists, paying for prescriptions, traveling to world-renowned doctors, etc.

Alternatively, where I live, a 30-minute visit with a naturopath or holistic dietician cost over $125.00. An hour of acupuncture from a good acupuncturist was $85.00. That is a lot of money to plunk down in one shot. I also had little faith they could possibly help me so why pay that much? After all, if a medical doctor who went to school for a gazillion years couldn't help me, how could a natural health practitioner?

To some degree it was true I needed the traditional doctors. Ultimately, major surgery did help me. However, natural practitioners helped me where traditional doctors could not. After the sphincteroplasty, my symptoms improved but I still had some lingering symptoms and now suffer from chronic pancreatitis. I currently utilize many different natural treatments for a variety of digestive symptoms and realized some natural practitioners were worth every penny they charged.

I know of many SOD patients who do well with natural treatments and almost never see a gastroenterologist or other specialist. The key is to keep trying things until you find what works. Today, naturopaths, functional medicine practitioners, and acupuncturists are my go-to health care providers before I head to the GI doctor. Or, I will figure something out on my own that works. I have definitely become quite the expert in researching treatments and pinpointing what could help me.

Just as natural treatments can be helpful, they can also harm. For example, I do not provide information about liver detoxes. They are commonly touted to clean the gallbladder out and rid the body of multiple gallstones, even "re-setting" the liver. They are harsh and put a great amount of stress on the liver and biliary system. In some instances, they can be beneficial, i.e. if you still get stones. Those with SOD may want to steer clear, though, as it could worsen the condition by putting more strain on the already strained organs and ducts.

Be especially cautious with supplements and herbs. For example, artichoke extract is supposed to help the liver and bile but it can also cause death if you have a biliary obstruction. Be cautious experimenting with "cures," especially if you don't know the exact cause of your symptoms.

Keep in mind, with almost every "remedy" you have to give it some time to see if it will help you. Doing anything once or twice and giving up on it is not what this is all about. Just the same if you wanted to see results from an exercise routine, you would need to practice every day. Nothing will magically happen overnight. Try different things and give each treatment some time to see if it will work. Be patient. I know it is easy for me to say this now. When I was at my sickest, every minute I was ill felt like an eternity.

The following treatments I am about to describe have been recommended by SOD patients or personally trialed by me. Before embarking on your natural remedy journey, I recommend you invest in a consult or two from one or more of the following practitioners:

Naturopathic Doctor—Treats patients using natural therapies such as physical manipulation, clinical nutrition, herbal medicine, homeopathy, counseling, acupuncture, and hydrotherapy. They choose treatments based on the individual patient, not based on the generality of symptoms. For some who prefer only a natural treatment route, they have made a naturopathic doctor their primary care physician.

Functional Medicine Doctor/Practitioner—Addresses the underlying causes of disease, engaging both patient and practitioner in a therapeutic partnership and individualized treatment plan. These practitioners address the whole person, not just an isolated set of symptoms, moving away from the traditional disease-centered focus of medical practice to a more patient-centered approach. These practitioners can be a medical doctor, nurse practitioner, pharmacist, chiropractor, or other licensed health professional who completed specialized training in this area of practice.

Chiropractor—Focuses on the diagnosis and treatment of neuromuscular disorders, with an emphasis on treatment through manual adjustment and/or manipulation of the spine. Today, many chiropractors are cross-trained in the same complimentary therapies naturopathic and functional medicine doctors practice.

Holistic Health Counselors and Nutritionists, Homeopaths, and Herbalists—Treat the whole person in the same manner as a naturopath or functional medicine practitioner but with less schooling. Relies mostly on homeopathic medicine, diet, herbs, and other natural remedies to treat the patient.

Supplements and Herbs

If you ever walked into a health food store or browsed an online supplement shop, you would agree picking out a supplement can be an overwhelming and confusing task. There are literally thousands of cure-alls to choose for any type of ailment. In the case of herbs and other supplements, I strongly recommend anyone with SOD see a naturopath, herbalist, or other qualified and preferably licensed natural health practitioner to not only prescribe supplements but also monitor you.

Your primary care doctor should be made aware of any supplements you take but keep in mind he or she may not approve of any supplements as they are not regulated like prescription and over the counter medications and many mainstream doctors are not open-minded or versed in supplements. At least that has been my experience.

In the end, be cautious and start slowly to see if you have a bad reaction. Just because it is "natural" does not mean it is safely indicated for someone with SOD or other health issues.

Magnesium

Many SOD patients say magnesium helps them as it has natural muscle relaxant qualities. Oral magnesium is fine but not if you have an issue with loose stools since magnesium is a natural laxative. If you tend to get constipated then magnesium may not only help your SOD symptoms but also get you going if you know what I mean. Alternatively, magnesium oil can be applied anywhere on the skin. I don't know how effective it is topically as studies vary. I used it topically for leg cramps and it worked great. Same goes for Epsom salt baths. A bath with a ¼ to ½ cup of Epsom salts is supposed to provide a good amount of magnesium through the skin. One woman with SOD gets magnesium injections and swears they have reduced the severity of her pain.

Valerian

Valerian is a herb with natural muscle relaxant/antispasmodic qualities. I prefer valerian tea or valerian that is "standardized" in a gel cap. Standardized means only the portion of a herb that is medicinal is used. Otherwise, if you buy something that is a whole herb you are getting the whole plant or root. For medicinal purposes, I like standardized versions of herbs. Be careful with valerian. It can make you drowsy. I have seen some extended release versions of valerian which may work better and reduce drowsiness as the herb is slowly absorbed by the body over a longer period of time.

Ginger

Ginger can be consumed as a tea, pickled, in candies, or the fresh root can be grated or juiced. Ginger has been used medicinally for thousands of years in India as a natural anti-inflammatory and anti-nausea food. *The Journal of Pain* reported about a research study that confirmed ginger was an effective natural anti-inflammatory that helped reduce pain and inflammation in test subjects, and in some instances topped NSAIDs like ibuprofen for pain relief. Ginger contains the 5-HT3 antagonists gingerols, shogaols, and galanolactone, giving it anti-nausea qualities.

Dandelion, Mustard Greens, and Beets

All of these are meant to support the liver and bile. All have liver and bile cleansing properties. I juice fresh organic dandelion leaves, mustard greens, and beets I get from the local food co-op.

Dandelion root can also be purchased as an herbal tea, supplement or concentrated tonic. Beets contain betaine and therefore are good for the liver and bile. Juicing beets is a great way to get a lot of good betaine in one gulp.

Probiotics

Probiotics are sometimes recommended by SOD patients. Our gut bacteria are like little mini engines controlling hormones, enzymes, metabolism, and who knows, maybe even our sphincters. Probiotics boost our body's supply of good bacteria and are believed to crowd out bad bacteria. I can't say if probiotics ever helped my SOD as I only took them to heal my gut after antibiotics. For that they were useful. I have tried numerous probiotics and found VSL 3 (http://www.vsl3.com/) to be the best for me. It is the most studied probiotic and can be ordered online or prescribed by a doctor. The downside is it is expensive, which seems to be the case for anything good for our health.

Bile Salts

SOD can cause bile to get backed up and not properly flow. This is a problem as we need bile to breakdown fats. If bile is not released at the time food needs it, intestinal problems and malabsorption can occur. Bile salts, primarily from ox bile, are available for purchase but should be taken with caution. Consult a natural health practitioner about the amount you should take.

Digestive Enzymes

There is a variety of over the counter digestive enzymes available to supplement the potential lack of enzymes produced by the pancreas. We need amylase, protease, and lipase, which are excreted by the pancreas, to digest everything—carbohydrates, proteins, and fats. If our pancreatic sphincter keeps closing, then we don't get enough of these enzymes. I prefer prescription enzymes but some people say they get relief from over the counter brands. I know a few vegetarians who won't take the prescription kind because they are made from pigs. Have a natural health practitioner recommend a brand.

Betaine HCL with Pepsin

I take betaine hydrochloride with pepsin to balance stomach acid especially when I have excess bile due to my SOD. Stomach acid is important for proper digestion and nutrient absorption and this supplement aids if you have low stomach acid. Bile acid is actually not an acid. It is more on the neutral or basic side of the ph scale. Therefore, if you are like me and had bile reflux from SOD, the bile is basically neutralizing the stomach acid. As I said, we need stomach acid, which is often contrary to popular belief. Researchers are now finding a whole host of problems with people who take acid reducing medications long term, including osteoporosis, mineral deficiencies, and dementia.

Betaine is also a substance that helps to protect the liver and stimulate the flow of bile. Pepsin is necessary for digesting proteins. I don't know how or why, but these supplements, when taken with meals, helped my nausea and improved my food sensitivities.

Bioidentical Hormones

These are not to be confused with prescription birth control. These are usually prescribed by a natural health practitioner and made at a compounding pharmacy. The practitioner will prescribe these based on symptomology or a blood and/or saliva hormone test. Progesterone, estrogen, DHEA, and testosterone are the most common of these hormones prescribed for replacement. Sometimes you can also acquire these creams already compounded. I wouldn't self-prescribe any hormone cream. You definitely want to get testing to ensure you are low in any of these hormones. I know a few women with SOD who said applying a compound of progesterone and estrogen or progesterone alone cured their SOD. They reported not having symptoms in years so long as they applied the cream daily.

Antioxidant Therapy for Chronic Pancreatitis

Many who have SOD also have chronic pancreatitis (CP) or end up having CP. Recently there have been quite a few studies focusing on antioxidant therapy. Some results have been promising while others inconclusive. It has been proposed there is a great deal of oxidative stress with CP and the antioxidants vitamin e and c, selenium, methionine, and flavonoids like those found in tea, grapeseed and resveratrol combat this. Also, individuals with CP tend to have low levels of these antioxidants in their blood. I started taking this last year. I am honestly not sure if they helped or not, but my functional medicine practitioner wants me to continue taking them so I will. That and I recently had a special blood nutrient test called Spectracell and coincidentally was deficient or low in all of these antioxidants.

Breathing and Meditation

Some may wonder how things like meditation and breathing help SOD. They help because the fact is that stress, anxiety, and depression impact our digestive system and pain perception. No, I am not insinuating SOD is all in your head. One of my biggest pet peeves is to hear about an SOD patient's health care provider suggesting their symptoms are psychological. That being said, though, stress and emotional imbalance could make things worse and impede recovery or remission. Therefore, it is important to treat our minds along with the rest of our bodies.

I can't tell you how many times I felt sick, then became stressed over being sick, then felt sicker because I was stressed, then felt more stressed because I was feeling sicker. This went on and on. It was a vicious cycle. Getting a handle on stress can help prevent SOD from spiraling out of control. Before my SOD became disabling, I led a productive, healthy, low-pain life with SOD for 12 years thanks to deep breathing exercises, meditation, yoga, diet, and lifestyle changes. You may never be completely rid of SOD pain or other symptoms, but these practices absolutely can help move them from the center stage of your life to the distant balcony.

Breathing

Breathing is so underrated. We do it several times during each minute of the day. In addition to sustaining our lives, amazing things happen on the cellular level when we breathe. Breathing deeply and with intention has shown to relieve stress and lessen pain.
Think about the popular childbirth breathing program, Lamaze. According to the Lamaze International website, conscious breathing (especially slow breathing) reduces heart rate, anxiety, and pain perception. It works in part because when breathing becomes a focus, other sensations, such as labor pain, move to the edge of your awareness. Conscious breathing also keeps the expectant mom and baby "well oxygenated."

Recently I came across a great article in *Yoga Journal* called, "The Science of Breathing." Fast uneven breathing triggers the nervous system, turning up stress hormones, heart rate, blood pressure, muscle tension, sweat production, and anxiety. Alternatively, slowing your breath dials down all of the above as it turns up relaxation, calm, and mental clarity. The deep inhales of conscious breathing introduce more oxygen into your body while deep release exhales remove the carbon dioxide waste products. In theory, more blood can be oxygenated using this technique.

So how does this help those with SOD? Well, aside from what I just wrote, I don't know. I do know that once I began practicing conscious breathing my pain was more manageable. The pain did not disappear. It became tolerable. Through my breathing practice, I was able to achieve a level of acceptance and patience around my painful condition. Prior to this, I was living in fight or flight mode, making the pain worse. Today, I continue to practice this type of breathing especially when stressed, worried or scared.

Conscious breathing is fairly simple. My only suggestion is to breathe deeply through your nose rather than your mouth. You will know you are doing it right when you make a slight hissing type sound, sort of like a light snore, at the base of your sinuses and beginning of your throat. Perform deep inhales for a count of at least four. You will want to fill your upper belly on inhale and deflate it on exhale. When inhaling, your goal is to stretch out your diaphragm, which serves as the main muscle of respiration and is attached to the lower ribs. Follow with an identical count exhale.

Meditation

For the longest time, I considered myself a meditation flunky. In vain, I have accumulated a rather large collection of books on meditation, including, "Meditation for Dummies" and viewed countless tutorials on how to meditate. Meditation alluded me for a very long time. Sitting still and quieting my mind was a constant struggle. Instead of clearing my head I would obsess over needing to vacuum the floor I was sitting on, or try to remember if I set the DVR for my favorite show. I would get uncomfortable sitting straight up. I'd slouch and readjust my leg fold to get comfortable, but to no avail.

Finally, I came to realize I was never going to be perfect at meditation and that was ok. I accepted the fact meditation was a lifelong work in progress. I changed my seated position to whatever position I felt comfortable, even if that meant lying down or curled up on the couch. I recognized the disruptive thoughts and imagined ushering them out of my psyche without judgment. "Goodbye thought," I'd say to myself. I started humming and incorporating my deep breathing. I still do not meditate perfectly or as often as would benefit me, but I'm doing my best and that's what matters.

Most days I take advantage of guided meditations to lead me to a place of peace. You can order guided meditations online. I prefer to search for free guided meditations on YouTube and listen to the videos. I also have a few meditation apps downloaded on my phone. Some people prefer podcasts. A few months ago I started attending group meditations at our city's local Buddhist center. They are an hour long and led by an experienced group meditation leader. The leader reads something then we meditate in a chair or on the floor for a half hour, followed by a slow walking meditation, and ending with a sitting meditation and a final reading. I started going because I knew if I went then I'd have to sit there and meditate. Sure enough, my theory worked.

Last year, I saw a certified hypnotist/hypnotherapist to strengthen my meditation practice and help me to cope with my chronic pancreatitis pain. It was very helpful. I still use some of the self-talk the therapist taught me to relax and focus on absolutely nothing.

Mindfulness Meditation—especially for eating

I have a friend who eats very slowly. Instead of getting annoyed over how long it would take her to finish her lunch or dinner, I admired the way she ate with such intention and care. She would savor every morsel of food as I inhaled a whole plate of food within minutes. I have always been a fast eater, someone who ate like it was their last meal. My dad would say I ate, "like it was going out of style."

With SOD I realized that overeating and stuffing my face made my symptoms worse. It put an incredible strain on organs already strained from the sphincters not working properly. I saw a naturopath who suggested a change in the way I ate. She called it, "food hygiene," and told me to chew my food 20 or more times and count as I chewed. I did this for a few weeks, then reverted back to my animalistic flare for eating. Recently I have come across something called "Mindful Eating." As I read about mindful eating I knew it was something I could benefit from doing. First, though, I educated myself on the practice of mindfulness.

I thought mindfulness and meditation were one and the same but they are a bit different. With mindfulness, you focus and set your intention on one thing. For example, this could be breathing, an object, imagined ball of color, or even a soothing word. This will lead you to a state of meditation in most instances. As in meditation, you get comfortable and acknowledge disruptive thoughts, then shoo them away. But with mindfulness, you are aware of your intention.

Your senses are highly alert. With breathing you would focus in on the air entering your nose and lungs, the smell of the air, the feeling of your lungs filling and diaphragm stretching. You would be in tune with whatever it is you are focusing on. You could replicate this exercise with, for example, the sun—sitting in the sun and feeling its warmth, brightness through your eyes. With words, you can say a soothing word repeatedly, like serenity, calm, or peace. Mindfulness is the ultimate practice for being present in the moment.

There are several books and websites dedicated to teaching you how to practice mindful eating. With mindful eating, you set your intention on the food you are about to eat. Take a piece of fruit. Hold it in your hand. I say a prayer of thanks for the food I am about to consume. Then hold the food to your nose and release your sense of smell. Eat the food slowly, moving it around your mouth. Notice the texture and taste. Chew slowly then swallow.

Make eating a process, rather than a shovel fest. You can incorporate counting your chews if you want. As long as your focus is on the slow process of acknowledging and engaging the food you eat. Many dietitians are touting mindfulness eating as a weight loss strategy. This may concern some of you who have unintentionally lost weight due to your SOD. I doubt you would lose much weight with mindfulness eating unless you also changed the food you were eating. Therefore, practicing it shouldn't detrimentally affect your weight.

Breathing and meditation are great, but I will be honest. On days when my pain flares, no amount of breathing or quieting the mind helps, which is good there are other "survival" techniques I can employ. Whether you utilize breathing and meditation as a complimentary treatment to your other SOD treatments or they are your only SOD treatment, I assure you will not be disappointed practicing these on a regular basis.

Yoga

I love yoga. I love yoga. I love yoga. Did I say I love yoga? Yoga is awesome, especially since it incorporates deep breathing throughout the poses. You can do yoga on your own or in a class environment. There are specific poses to regenerate and relax the digestive system. I strongly recommend learning in a beginner's class before embarking on your own. This way you can be assured your posture is correct so you don't injure yourself. You want to be sure you are benefiting from the poses, not making matters worse. Also, a local yoga teacher may have tips for poses that will help your SOD.

Yoga is offered in yoga studios, churches, community centers and many other places. I even did something called Hiking Yoga in Central Park, New York. Today I stick to yoga classes at the gym I belong. They have yoga class offerings nearly every day with a variety of teachers. There are definitely certain yoga teachers I prefer over others. Keep trying different classes until you find one you like.

I also get the mat out and do a series of poses on my own at home. I own several yoga DVDs and still use one meant for pregnancy from five years ago as I like the yoga teacher's demeanor and choice of poses. I also own one specifically meant for people with digestive issues. I generally steer clear of hardcore yoga DVDs meant for weight loss. It kind of defeats the purpose of yoga if the yoga teacher is yelling at me to "feel the burn."

You can find a plethora of free yoga tutorials on YouTube and the Internet. Search using terms like, "yoga for the digestive system" or "relaxing yoga". There is no shortage of information on yoga poses for digestion. However, I haven't come across any poses specifically for SOD. To get more specific, you could also search the Internet for "yoga poses for the liver" or "yoga poses for the pancreas."

I have been doing yoga as long as I have had SOD—around 17 years as of this writing. Yoga is a wonderful tool for grounding, relaxation, meditating, deep breathing and strengthening the muscles surrounding our testy little sphincter of Oddi.

Tai Chi, Qi Gong

Tai chi is a centuries-old Chinese martial art that descends from qigong, an ancient Chinese discipline that has its roots in traditional Chinese medicine. You may have seen people moving gracefully with flowing motions in parks doing Tai Chi. The core training involves two primary features: the first being taolu (solo "forms"), a slow sequence of movements which emphasize a straight spine, abdominal breathing and a natural range of motion; the second being different styles of tuishou ("pushing hands") for training movement principles of the form with a partner and in a more practical manner. Some SOD patients have reported benefits from practicing Tai Chi.

Acupuncture

I tried acupuncture numerous times. It was a miracle cure for my third pregnancy morning sickness. It helped minimally, though, for my SOD symptoms. The thing with acupuncture is you definitely have to go consistently. The best results I experienced were when I went twice a week. This became very expensive but I did find a place that offered community acupuncture for half the price. Community acupuncture is where you get acupuncture in the same room as a few other people. I learned quickly to bring my headphones to listen to soft music, as a few of the other patients snored.

According to the *Gastrointestinal Endoscopy* article, "Electroacupuncture May Relax the Contraction of Sphincter of Oddi", electroacupuncture stimulation of acupoint GB 34 resulted in reversible inhibition of sphincter of Oddi contraction in humans. If you see an acupuncturist be sure to let them know about this fact.

Essential Oils

Some people I know swear by using essential oils for just about every ailment. A dot of an essential oil (they are concentrated and strong) is generally applied to the feet or belly area. You can also add a couple drops to a carrier oil like olive oil, avocado oil, or my favorite combination—organic wheat germ and jojoba oil. I recommend buying organic essential and carrier oils where the herbs and soil were not sprayed with pesticides.

Go slow with essential oils and be cautious. Essential oils seem innocent but can be potent and cause reactions in some people. There are many Internet resources available for researching which oils help with what ailments. Search for these essential oil qualities: antispasmodic, anti-nausea, anti-inflammatory and digestive.

Ayurveda

Ayurveda is a 5,000-year-old system of natural healing from India. It relies on multiple regimens to attain health and includes building a healthy metabolic system and maintaining good digestion and excretion, lifestyle, yoga, meditation, life-affirming mental attitude, therapies as well as Ayurvedic medicine. Ayurvedic professionals use the five senses to diagnose and some therapies rely on herbal compounds. To find an Ayurveda professional, you can search on the Internet or call local holistic wellness and naturopathic centers.

Castor Oil Packs

The first naturopath I saw recommended I apply castor oil packs daily for my SOD symptoms. It didn't help me all that much but I figured I would put it in here as some people say it helped their digestive symptoms. The reported medicinal uses of castor oil packs are: drawing impurities from the liver, improving circulation, draining the lymphatic system, and combatting inflammation.

This is how I made my castor oil pack: Cut a piece of flannel so it is big enough to cover your right upper quadrant (half of the front part of your abdomen and half of the back around the right ribs). Drench the flannel in a high-grade non-toxic brand of castor oil. Apply the flannel to the right upper quadrant and wrap saran plastic wrap around your torso and the flannel to hold it in place and keep it covered and protected.

Apply a large heating pad to the entire area. I will be honest that it is a very relaxing treatment. So, whether it truly can heal SOD, at least you will be relaxed and your skin smoother. One word of caution is not to use castor oil packs if you are pregnant, as castor oil is reported to induce labor.

Biofeedback

This type of therapy is typically done with a mental health therapist but can be self-administered through computer programs. During a biofeedback session, electrodes are attached to your skin which record your heart and breathing rate, blood pressure, skin temperature, sweating, and/or muscle activity. When you are under stress or experience pain, it will show on the monitor. A biofeedback therapist, or the computer program, will help you practice relaxation exercises, which will be practiced to coincide with monitoring your different bodily functions with the goal of pain and stress relief, and wellbeing.

Reiki

Reiki is based on qi ("chi"), a life energy/force that is reported to exist within us. It is a form of hands-on-healing. The reiki practitioner transfers their positive energy to the recipient which encourages healing. Reiki addresses physical, emotional, mental, and spiritual imbalances. Up until a year ago, I thought reiki was ridiculously fake and hokey. In 2012, I had reiki performed on me by volunteers in the hospital and felt no better or worse. Last year I had several reiki sessions and every time, at the end of the treatment, I'd feel a shift in my energy level and cried for no reason other than it was cleansing. As the day went on, my pancreatic pain lessened. Now I don't know what to think. Our local food co-op has reiki volunteers who donate their time so it was free for me to sign up for a ½ hour session. Even if it is nothing but a placebo effect, at least I felt better after each session.

Visceral massage

Massage that targets the area between the skin, muscles, and internal organs, sometimes actually massaging the organ (externally of course) is called visceral massage. Some SOD patients have had visceral massage sessions targeting the sphincter of Oddi area and say it helped. It is believed non-muscular organs like the kidneys, liver, stomach, intestines, pancreas, etc. can harden and inhibit blood flow. It is also thought organs can form trigger points, which are thought to be points of local tenderness to broader areas, referring pain and/or tension elsewhere. Visceral massage is often used to heal adhesions (scar tissue) deeply embedded around a surgical area that may have spread.

Chapter 7: SOD Diet

Quite often I am asked whether there is a special diet for SOD; and my answer is always the same, "No." There is no perfect SOD diet because each SOD patient is different. Some foods triggering one person's symptoms may be a safe food for someone else. There also exists a uniqueness between people with biliary and pancreatic issues and their tolerance of certain foods. Keep in mind, there are three sphincter areas that can dysfunction. Some people have an issue with one sphincter area while others have a problem with all three. That is why some experience biliary symptoms while others lean to pancreatic symptoms and yet others experience both biliary and pancreatic symptoms.

All that being said, this does not mean there aren't dietary guidelines or practices that could benefit a person with SOD. It is well-documented food plays a role in pain attacks and the severity and frequency of other symptoms. There are also varying degrees of SOD. Some patients can eat anything and experience only occasional pain. Others have trouble with everything they ingest, leaving them with severe unrelenting pain, nausea, vomiting, unintended weight loss, diarrhea and/or constipation.

Food Diary and Elimination Diet

The first step to finding the nutritional plan best suited for you is with a food and symptom diary. Food diaries are easy tools to identify trigger and safe foods. There is no hard rule of what this diary should look like but a good food and symptom diary is broken down by daily time intervals like morning, mid-morning, noon, afternoon, evening, and late evening. You may keep notes in a notebook, on your computer, or in your phone.

In fact, there are a variety of free or affordable food diary apps for your phone or tablet you can download. Whatever form of a food diary you decide upon doesn't matter as long as you are diligent in recording everything you put in your mouth, i.e. food, beverages, supplements and medications; and the symptoms you feel throughout the day. This will help you identify what is safe and not safe to consume. Activities like exercise or meditation should also be included.

The food diary doesn't just isolate foods as they affect you. Absolutely anything you ingest is fair game to affect your SOD. Seemingly innocent vitamins, minerals, herbal supplements, and medications can be triggers. I figured out certain brands of valerian actually made my SOD flare once it started wearing off, though it helped for the first hour after taking it.

I have allergies and found if I ingested certain herbal teas like chamomile I'd get stomach cramps and headaches. This made sense because I have seasonal allergies and chamomile is a herb. In other words, if I was allergic to breathing in a plant, then, of course, my body would react to ingesting it. I know this isn't an SOD issue but it was interesting to find out things like sensitivities and intolerances while in the pursuit of SOD triggers.

Beverages could also be an issue. I would develop severe SOD pain after drinking carbonated drinks like soda or seltzer. I tried changing soda brands and flavors, thinking it was the artificial flavorings, colorings or sweeteners of a particular brand. I soon discovered soda, even sparkling water and my beloved kombucha tea, caused pain and concluded it was the carbonation not the ingredients which caused the problem. My theory was the air from the carbonation got "stuck" in the ducts as the sphincters spasm open and shut, causing pressure and pain.

Deducing the origin of SOD triggers takes investigative work and patience. Some food reactions may be instant while others are delayed. You may experience a symptom from a food several hours after ingesting and confuse the reaction with a food you ate later on. For this reason, I recommend starting your food diary with a strict food elimination plan then slowly reintroduce the foods and treats you like. Foods with multiple ingredients should be kept to a minimum.

For example, I know many SOD patients who react to mashed potatoes. The problem with mashed potatoes is there are several ingredients which could cause the problem, i.e. potatoes, milk, butter, seasonings, etc. If you had a plain potato and it didn't bother you but mashed potatoes did, then undoubtedly you are sensitive to the dairy or the fat content of the added ingredients. Even an otherwise innocent seasoning could be to blame. I couldn't touch onion or garlic products—even a dash—without having an attack. I have no idea why this happened but it was extremely difficult, especially at restaurants, to get food that wasn't seasoned with them. On top of it, wait staff never got it right when assuring me these seasonings weren't in a dish I'd ordered.

Most elimination diets are meant to identify allergies or food sensitivities. SOD triggers are not allergies per se, but SOD may lead to food sensitivities or intolerances especially if bile and pancreatic enzyme output are impeded. Most food elimination plans will recommend eliminating the most common food allergy/sensitivity offenders like dairy, nuts, soy, eggs, peanuts, gluten, etc. You can do this, but from my experience, SOD is not typically triggered by a food allergy or sensitivity. The key is keeping it simple in the beginning to foods like rice, lean meat, vegetables, and some fruits. At the very least, eliminate the most commonly reported SOD triggers. Some of these are:

Coffee and anything with caffeine
Chocolate
Red meat and pork, even lean cuts
Fried foods
Spicy foods
Fatty and oily foods
Alcohol
Some fruits especially acidic fruits
Difficult to digest raw vegetables

You may also want to try removing any foods with a high nitrate content. Since it has been said nitrates decrease the resistance offered by the sphincter, eliminate them to see if you aren't experiencing some weird rebound effect from eating them. I am reaching for straws here and have no proof high nitrate foods are detrimental. However, it doesn't hurt to include them in the food elimination trials. You don't have to eliminate all of them forever.

Foods potentially high in nitrates are lunch meat, beef or other types of jerky, sausages, and hot dogs. Look out for anything labeled "cured" (you could eat them if they say "nitrate-free"). Other foods naturally high in nitrates are non-organic fruits and vegetables (these often come into contact with nitrate-rich fertilizer), root vegetables like carrots and potatoes, spinach, broccoli, cauliflower; and well water (try to drink bottled or jugs of spring or purified water).

Avoid anything high in monosodium glutamate (MSG) or additives resembling glutamic acid. These can be excitatory to the nervous system. Since we don't know the exact neural component to SOD, it's best to try eliminating them. If you eat Chinese takeout be sure to tell them not to add any MSG. Many restaurant items have MSG so ask. There is glutamate hidden everywhere. As of this writing, the website, http://www.truthinlabeling.org/hiddensources.html, lists more than 40 different ingredients containing the chemical in MSG (processed free glutamic acid).

Track your symptoms and within a few days try to reintroduce foods one at a time. Have a good amount of the food so you can see if it causes symptoms. Continue to add back foods one at a time every few days. If symptoms don't make your SOD symptoms flare, keep that food in your ongoing diet. Anything that causes a flare up should be eliminated. After a week or two try adding it back again. If again it causes a flare up, eliminate it for good from your diet.

Juicing and Blending

Many SOD patients report feeling better when they juice or eat a blended diet. You may want to stick to juicing and blending during your food elimination stage. Juicing and blending are different but similar. Both make it easier for your body to absorb nutrients as they are in the form of micronutrients. A juiced vegetable may take less than 30 minutes to digest while its raw whole counterpart could take 6 hours or more. Juicing vegetables and fruits with a juicer (not to be confused with an extractor) squeezes juice from the food. None of the fibers or proteins are included in the juice extract and nutrients are more easily and quickly absorbed.

Blending or extracting (think Ninja or Vitamix appliance) emulsifies the vegetable or fruit, leaving the juice and fibers intact. For some people, this can be an issue as it is very high in fiber. A high fiber diet is contraindicated for people with certain intestinal conditions and those with post-gallbladder diarrhea. If you are someone who does better with extra fiber, then this may be the way to go but for those sensitive to high fiber diets, you may want to stick with juicing.

I recommend homemade blended smoothies before drinking preservative- and artificial ingredient-laden drinks like Ensure or Muscle Milk. You can make smoothies with any kind of pure protein powder. Whey is a popular protein powder. I buy undenatured organic whey as it is purer and less processed. Rice, pea or hemp protein powder are good choices as well but may be grittier. The only protein I don't recommend is soy protein.

Soy can be inflammatory for many people. The last thing a person with SOD needs to ingest is something that will cause inflammation. Soy is one of my trigger foods so I avoid it entirely. Some people who can't tolerate regular soy do ok with fermented soy products. The other issue with soy is that most soy products are a genetically modified organism (GMO) food product, which I'll talk about in the next paragraph.

Once you have selected a protein powder, put a few scoops in a blender and add vegetables and fruits and/or their juice, yogurt or kefir (a yogurt drink) if you want, and a healthy fat like flax or olive oil (warning: even healthy oils/fats can cause an SOD flare so test it out). It isn't fun to live on a liquid diet but can be useful during severe flare-ups as a meal replacement. There are also good medical food replacement supplements. They are advertised as meal replacements and some as leaky gut supplements. They are usually made with rice protein. As of this writing, there is one called GI Sustain by Metagenics (http://www.metagenics.com/mp/medical-foods/gi-sustain). I don't have a stake in the company or product. I just know some people with unintended weight loss and malabsorption issues who benefited from it.

Good Diet Habits

Eat organic and non-processed foods. Ideally, shop in the outer aisles of the grocery store. I particularly steer clear of GMO foods, which are engineered to withstand large applications of Roundup, a toxic fertilizer. GMO foods aren't the same foods our ancestors ate, which could mean they are harder to digest. I also advocate consuming only antibiotic-free meat. The antibiotics injected into these animals are often powerful and can be neurotoxic.

Quite often the meat industry uses fluoroquinolone antibiotics which were invented to kill Anthrax! These antibiotics end up in our bodies, disrupting our precious microbiome. Your liver will love you for keeping your diet clean as it has to work overtime to detoxify foods containing pesticides, preservatives, artificial flavorings and coloring and other toxins.

The liver experiences a great deal of strain already when the sphincter continuously spasms shut, causing bile to backup. When we flood our bodies with toxic substances, our liver, pancreas and intestines have to work extra hard to remove them from the body. Ideally, bile acts as a detergent to break down fats and carry toxins out of the body.

However, not all bile is excreted and instead is reabsorbed by the intestine and sent back to the liver. These toxins can end up back in the liver where it joins more toxins accumulated from the present. The more work the liver has to do the more stress to the biliary system and possibly the sphincters. Stay away from high fructose corn syrup too as it is the leading contributor to fatty liver disease. Many SOD patients report having a fatty liver show up on their scans. I did.

Specific Diets

Some report benefiting from specific diets, the most common being anything low fat. I have several low-fat cookbooks on my computer tablet so meals don't get boring and I don't feel deprived. I don't think anyone with SOD can go wrong with a low-fat diet. Some find it helpful to count fat grams and keep it under a certain amount as determined by their food diary. One popular diet my gastroenterologists and dieticians recommended was the FODMAP diet. It is usually reserved for irritable bowel syndrome, but some with SOD and chronic pancreatitis say it helped them.

FODMAP stands for Fermentable Oligosaccharides, Disaccharides, Monosaccharides, and Polyols. These foods contain difficult-to-digest sugars and fibers that can cause bowel problems like excess gas, painful bloating, and constipation or diarrhea. You can do an Internet search for FODMAP. You will find many different websites on this topic along with lists of which foods to avoid and which are safe foods. As of this writing, I found that dietician Kate Scarlata's website (http://www.katescarlata.com/) provided the most comprehensive information on FODMAPs.

Examples of common foods to avoid are wheat, onion, garlic, beans, apples, lactose-containing dairy, and high fructose sweeteners. FODMAPs is restrictive, but for my pancreatic symptoms, it has been very helpful. I believe when I eat FODMAPs, the resulting excess gas gets trapped in the biliary or pancreatic duct due to the faulty sphincters, causing pain. When I do eat a FODMAP item I am sure to take an activated charcoal capsule after the meal to "mop up" the gas.

Another diet strategy many people with SOD employ is to go gluten free. Gluten is a protein present in many grains, particularly wheat, that is linked to a serious intestinal disease called celiac disease. It is also linked to leaky gut, which is another way of saying the small intestine's lining is damaged. Gluten free is a big craze now but I am yet to meet anyone whose SOD symptoms were completely relieved by going gluten free. Some do report feeling better having gone gluten free but it is likely these people have celiac disease or a gluten sensitivity. Going gluten free is not a panacea for curing your SOD.

In fact, there are a lot of gluten-free items with nasty ingredients that could trigger SOD symptoms. When my SOD was at its worst I went gluten-free for a whole year. I was strict about it and felt no better or worse. I personally do not believe gluten is entirely evil, but I do make an effort to limit the amount of gluten I eat in a week. If I do eat something with gluten in it, I focus more on staying away from GMO wheat/grains. There is certainly no harm in trying a gluten free lifestyle. Just stick with whole foods and not gluten free items loaded with ingredients you can't pronounce.

Food Combining

With SOD we want to make digestion as easy a process as possible. Food combining can accomplish this. Eating some food groups together can be a disaster for your digestive system. Food combining enthusiasts recommend never eating a heavy protein with a heavy carbohydrate or starch. In other words, eating meat and a potato is a no no. Same goes for meat with pasta or bread. Instead, eat meats, beans, or tofu with a non-starchy vegetable. The same goes for eating a heavy carbohydrate. Pair it with a non-starchy vegetable.

Avoid large amounts of fat with protein, like the extra mayonnaise in a chicken salad or olive oil drizzled on a chicken breast, because it slows digestion. This is one of the reasons pizza is an SOD nightmare food. You've got all of the big offenders: heavy fatty protein (cheese) and heavy carbohydrate high FODMAP (wheat pizza dough). The tomato sauce is likely ok unless it has a high amount of onions and garlic which are high in FODMAPs. I love pizza but it never failed. If I took even a few bites, I'd have a pain attack. As for fruit, eat fruit alone, on an empty stomach.

Final Words on Diet

In closing, I think it is fitting I mention that one of my worst triggers was going too long without eating. Yes, *not* eating triggered SOD pain. I thought I was alone with this issue until others agreed this happened to them too. It was like the stress of being hungry caused pain. The other extreme, overeating, was a trigger too. Overeating puts stress on all of the organs and the sphincters. It's best to eat small frequent meals. Chewing thoroughly and slowly will benefit your entire digestive tract and organs so they don't have to work as hard. Your digestive system starts in your mouth where enzymes are released to start the digestion process.

Chapter 8: Medications

Medications can be beneficial for alleviating SOD symptoms like pain and nausea in some people. The first course of treatment a physician commonly takes for SOD relief, after diet and lifestyle modifications fail, is prescribing a medication. Ideally, doctors would exhaust all medication options before advancing to an invasive treatment option.

Throughout my participation in SOD groups, I have witnessed profound variations regarding medication success with each individual patient. One woman will tell you she gets complete relief from a calcium channel blocker, antispasmodic, or other medication while these same medications offer no relief for others with the same condition. Some tolerate side effects while others cannot get past a single dose. This can be a problem when a high dose of a medication is required to have an effect on the sphincters. It is unfortunate to witness an SOD patient find relief in a medication then have to cease taking it because the side effects became worse than the actual SOD.

The following is a description of the most commonly prescribed medications for SOD symptoms. I mostly used the United States generic drug names. If you are from a different country, you should easily be able to find their counterparts by searching online. This is by no means a complete list. It is likely with new drugs always on the horizon and others not available in the U.S. or in other countries, I may have unintentionally omitted effective drugs. This list was compiled from SOD patient surveys, support group input and research articles.

There are medications for almost every digestive condition. Although many people with SOD also have other co-occurring digestive issues like ulcerative colitis, Crohn's disease, acid reflux, irritable bowel syndrome, and small intestinal bacterial overgrowth to name a few, I will focus on medications targeting common SOD symptoms rather than include those for all digestive disorders.

Anticholinergics and Antispasmodics

Anticholinergics interfere with the action of the neurochemical acetylcholine and block involuntary movements. They stop the transmission of parasympathetic nerve impulses, therefore, lessening the spasms of smooth muscle, such as in the gastrointestinal tract and in the bladder. Most antispasmodic agents are also anticholinergics. They can work directly on the smooth muscle in the wall of the gut. Here they help to relax the muscle and relieve the pain associated with a contraction of the gut.

Since the sphincter of Oddi is a tiny smooth muscle it is thought this class of drugs will prevent the sphincter from spasm and quell the nerve pain associated with SOD. I have witnessed many SOD sufferers gain relief by taking this class of drugs. In addition to SOD pain, these drugs may be prescribed for biliary colic (spasm) and nausea. Side effects are generally minimal, but for some become intolerable. The most common are mucous membrane dryness, dizziness, and drowsiness.

Examples of anticholinergic/antispasmodic agents are hyoscyamine, chlordiazepoxide/clidinium, dicyclomine, scopolamine, glycopyrrolate, amitriptyline, nortriptyline, atropine, mebeverine (not available in the U.S.), and combos of these generics with phenobarbital and belladonna.

Muscle Relaxants

Muscle relaxants are agents that reduce tension in muscles. Centrally acting muscle relaxants work by reducing the tone of skeletal muscle causing muscles to relax. These are generally used to relieve skeletal muscle spasms due to spastic conditions, and can be used to relieve musculoskeletal pain. Some muscle relaxers also work by blocking pain sensations between the nerves and the brain.

Like with the anticholinergic/antispasmodic class of drugs, muscle relaxants are prescribed to stop the sphincter of Oddi from spasm and help control the pain related to this tiny little muscle. An interesting observation is the people I know who gained relief from muscle relaxants also got relief from biliary stents and the biliary roux en y surgery, leading me to believe these individuals had issues solely with their biliary sphincter and/or bile duct and not the pancreatic sphincter.

Examples of muscle relaxers are cyclobenzaprine, carisoprodol, baclofen, and buscopan. Common side effects are similar to anticholinergics and antispasmodics.

Calcium Channel Blockers

Calcium channel blockers are typically used to treat high blood pressure and heart conditions. They act as a smooth muscle selective calcium channel antagonists and potent inhibitors of sphincter of Oddi contractions. This medication is particularly helpful when a patient is having a painful attack. The downside is its effect on blood pressure. If someone has low or even normal blood pressure, these medications can cause a severe drop in blood pressure. If you do not have low blood pressure and experience sudden pain attacks, you may want to discuss this medication with your doctor. Examples of calcium channel blockers are nitroglycerin, nifedipine, diltiazem, amlodipine, and felodipine.

Anti-epileptic Anticonvulsant Medication

This class of drugs was created to mimic some of the effects of GABA, an inhibitory neurotransmitter found in the central nervous system (CNS) that regulates its excitability. These drugs are used with other medications to prevent and control seizures. It is also used to relieve nerve pain. Some gastroenterologists believe SOD pain is a neuralgia, which is pain from damaged nerves. Drugs in this class most often prescribed for SOD are gabapentin and pregabalin. Both drugs can make you drowsy. Reviews are mixed on these for SOD—about half and half. I've heard more success stories with pregabalin.

Anti-nausea (Antiemetic) Medications

Anti-nausea/Antiemetic medications are used to control nausea and vomiting. If nausea and vomiting are uncontrollable, oral therapy may not be appropriate and intravenous or suppository administration at a hospital may be necessary. The first type of anti-nausea/antiemetic medication is the 5-HT3 receptor antagonist, which blocks serotonin receptors in the central nervous system and gastrointestinal tract.

The most common 5-HT3 receptor antagonist prescribed for nausea is ondansetron. This drug was once reserved for cancer patients receiving chemotherapy but is now widely used for any type of nausea syndrome, including morning sickness during pregnancy. It is most useful because it is non-sedating. Mirtazapine is another example, but it is quite sedating and prescribed mostly as an antidepressant.

The second type of anti-nausea/antiemetic are the dopamine antagonists, which block dopamine receptors. The most commonly prescribed in this class are metoclopramide and domperidone. These are also pro-kinetics, which increase gut motility and can help alleviate symptoms of gastroparesis (slow gut motility). It baffles me that domperidone is not FDA approved in the U.S. but metoclopramide is. Some of metoclopramide's side effects are serious and dangerous, including tardive dyskinesia, irregular blood pressure, and neuroleptic disorders. There are a few SOD patients who say they take it with no side effects. Just be very careful with it and alert your doctor of any strange effects.

Domperidone has not been approved here because it caused some heart irregularities in those receiving it intravenously in very large amounts. It also raises levels of the hormone prolactin which is why some use it to increase breast milk supply. Prolactin triggers milk production but high prolactin levels have been linked to pituitary gland tumors. In the U.S., domperidone can be acquired by prescription if made by a compounding pharmacy. There are also several websites where it can be ordered overseas, as it can be purchased over the counter in most other countries.

My domperidone was prescribed by a local GI doctor but it was too costly to purchase through a compounding pharmacy. All I will say is I got my domperidone one way or another. I thanked God every day I had it on hand when I needed it. The only side effect I experienced was an increase in my neuropathy. During periods when I took it regularly I had my prolactin levels monitored by my doctor. It has been a miracle drug for my nausea.

Antihistamines (H1 histamine receptor antagonists) are used off-label for nausea and vomiting but carry drowsiness as a side effect. Most antihistamines can be purchased over the counter like diphenhydramine, meclizine, and dimenhydrinate. The more sedating brands require a prescription, ex. promethazine and hydroxyzine.

Bile Medications

Many with SOD have bile reflux and biliary sludge issues. Bile reflux occurs when bile refluxes up into the stomach causing burning pain and nausea. Many doctors prescribe proton pump inhibitors (PPIs) or acid reducers, which are indicated for acid reflux or excess stomach acid. Bile reflux is completely different from acid reflux. PPIs aren't appropriate for bile reflux as it stops the overactive release of stomach acid. Theoretically, they wouldn't have an effect on refluxed bile acid. In addition, when bile enters the stomach it naturally reduces the acidity of stomach acid. Like I mentioned earlier, you want a good amount of stomach acid to properly digest proteins and metabolize certain vitamins and minerals.

Cholestyramine is a helpful medication for bile reflux as it binds to bile and carries it out of the body through the feces. It is usually prescribed for bile acid diarrhea, a well-documented problem for people with post-gallbladder issues like SOD. Cholestyramine is gritty and doesn't taste all that great, but it is an effective drug for those with severe bile acid issues. People with high cholesterol will benefit from this drug as it also lowers blood cholesterol levels.

I will never forget seeing a YouTube video about a reporter from England who had SOD. He had most of the markers for SOD Type 1 and the added bonus of acute pancreatitis episodes. For a long time, nothing helped—no medications, procedures, or natural remedies. One day his doctor prescribed cholestyramine. He has been well ever since.

Another medication which may help is sucralfate. Sucralfate is chalky and mops up acids. It is meant for short term use. Those with Lyme disease and similar syndromes must know that sucralfate contains aluminum and could have difficulty expelling it. Over the counter antacids containing calcium may help with bile reflux too as it can bind bile.

Biliary sludge seems to be a common issue for people with SOD. Bile becomes thick and sludge-like when it develops microscopic gallstone crystals. No one knows exactly why this happens, but for those without a gallbladder, it could be the result of bile not flowing properly. Also, when the sphincters spasm and stay shut for long periods, bile gets backed up. Ursodeoxycholic acid may be used to dissolve these microscopic gallstones and "thin" the bile. It is the only FDA-approved drug to treat primary biliary cirrhosis.

Prescription Pancreatic Enzymes

When my SOD became horribly problematic after the birth of my third son I developed a whole cadre of new SOD symptoms. One that was horribly painful originated from the pancreas. I didn't think anything could be worse than SOD pain until I experienced pancreatic pain. I suffered without treatment for six months before a GI doctor finally thought maybe prescribed enzymes (pancrealipase) would be helpful. A week after taking my first pill the pain was nearly gone. I still take them and still have pancreatic pain, but the enzymes help and also help me absorb food.

Medical Marijuana

I know many people with SOD who say they wouldn't be able to work or function if not for marijuana or marijuana derivatives. They laud its miraculous ability to improve pain, nausea, anxiety, stress, etc. The problem is it isn't legal everywhere so the pot you just purchased from your brother in law's "connection" may not be an appropriate strain for your SOD symptoms. If you purchase it as medical marijuana or in a legal state, your chances of obtaining a "perfect match" strain for your symptoms increases dramatically. I wouldn't attempt to recommend a strain and will leave that up to the experts. The only suggestion I can give you is if you use marijuana medicinally, be careful ingesting it as it could exacerbate your digestive issues. Vaporizing or using an oil or tincture may be the best option.

Opioid Pain Medication

Most opioid pain medications carry "spasm of sphincter of Oddi" as a side effect. Some, though, are definitely worse than others. As I mentioned previously, morphine was used for several decades to test for SOD spasm, so you may want to stay away from that one. Other opioid pain medication may exacerbate the spasm but most SOD patients I know seem to do ok with oxycodone, hydrocodone, fentanyl (in the form of patches), or hydromorphone if taken on occasion. Meperidine (Demerol) may be the best analgesic for hospitalized SOD patients. A study of 47 patients showed meperidine did not alter sphincter pressures in manometry patients.

Opioid pain medication is meant for acute pain and short term use. However, anyone who has had a severe chronic pain condition like SOD knows that may not be realistic and opioid treatment difficult to obtain. There are several dilemmas these drugs present, including their addictive nature (and subsequent withdrawal syndrome), the opiophobic trend of doctors, and criminalization of these drugs. The SOD patients I know who rely on pain medication and are successful in their use of it are closely monitored by a pain management doctor. They are routinely drug tested and allotted a certain amount so they do not abuse the drugs.

Unfortunately, in today's day and age most SOD patients are treated as drug seekers or refused pain management as they do not have something life threatening like cancer. SOD is poorly understood by most pain doctors. They cannot grasp that SOD could possibly be as painful as cancer pain and in some cases more painful.

It frustrates me to no end when I read countless stories of SOD patients using the emergency room as their pain management solution because they have been abandoned or ignored by their own doctors. There are many times my pain was extremely high on the 0 to 10 pain scale and no doctor would help to manage the pain. They all seemed to think the pain couldn't be that bad and to just live with it. At one point a GI doctor I later fired said it didn't matter I was in that much pain. They would tell me opioid pain medication would make it worse.

But in the cases I was medicated it made it better so who was right? Many pain management doctors where I live will not prescribe pain medication under any circumstances, which does leave it up to hospital emergency rooms to act as pain management programs. Instead, the trend is pain doctors push injections and spinal cord stimulators, which carry their own risk, aren't evidence-based for SOD, and are invasive.

I don't know what the solution is other than to encourage SOD patients to seek treatment when it gets bad enough. If your doctors won't prescribe anything, try everything else to relieve the pain. If that does not work, please head to an emergency room, though some are moving away from treating pain. If you are prescribed opioid pain medication, take as minimal a dose as possible, but work with your doctor on determining what that is. I have seen too many SOD patients build up a tolerance to pain medication to the point their doctors don't feel comfortable prescribing the amount they are on. Also, when tolerance is too high and you go into a flare, intravenous doses of pain medication administered in the hospital may not get the pain under control.

Naloxone/Naltrexone

Naloxone, an opiate blocker used to treat opioid overdoses, and as an opioid withdrawal aid has been shown to reverse opioid-induced sphincter of Oddi spasms. There are, though, only a few case studies about this and those studies were based on opioid-dependent patients. It is hard to say if the naloxone itself reduced SOD spams or if it was because the naloxone was administered to counteract opioids, hence stopping opioid-induced sphincter of Oddi spasms. It certainly is a drug worthy of future studies. A few SOD patients in our support group reported getting pain relief from low dose naltrexone, also an opiate blocker, which patients in the U.S. must acquire from a compounding pharmacy. High doses of naltrexone are given in pill form or as a monthly shot to counteract the effects of opioids. In other words, addicts on these drugs will not get high if they ingest opioids.

Benzodiazepines

According to the *National Library of Medicine,* benzodiazepines are a large class of medications that have multiple clinical uses including therapy of anxiety, insomnia, muscle spasm, alcohol withdrawal, and seizures. The pharmacological effects of the benzodiazepines are a result of their interaction with the central nervous system, their effects being sedation, hypnosis, decreased anxiety, muscle relaxation, anterograde amnesia and anticonvulsant activity.

Benzodiazepines can be very useful drugs for SOD nausea, vomiting, dizziness, and to ameliorate the stress and anxiety associated with this syndrome. Sounds like a wonder drug, right? Let me tell you they are not. The downside is benzodiazepines are highly addictive. Meaning, they are a bitch to come off if you've been on them a while. And, your tolerance can build up so you require more and more. The horror stories of interdose withdrawal and withdrawal syndrome are prevalent on the Internet. These drugs are best used for short periods or on occasion. In fact, it is widely documented that these medications are not recommended beyond a few weeks.

If it weren't for the temporary use of benzodiazepines when my SOD disabled me, I would have lost my mind. The most useful aspect was its effect on my nausea and vomiting. The benzodiazepine did not cure my SOD nausea but it did alleviate the intense anxiety and "out of control" feeling severe nausea inflicted. 24/7 nausea for a few days would make even the sanest person lose their mind. Mine was never-ending. I'd wake up with nausea, get anxiety about it, which brought on more nausea, which then brought on more anxiety. It was a vicious cycle.

Unfortunately, like with most benzos, my body became dependent. It was hell coming off of them and in the end I believe this class of drugs was to blame for pancreatic flares years after my sphincteroplasty. Yes, coming off medications can produce side effects just as bad or worse than the actual drug can. I have met many people on the Internet, particularly the Benzo Buddies website (http://www.benzobuddies.org), who developed SOD and pancreatic symptoms around the time they started on a benzo, tapered off, or went "cold turkey" abruptly.

Birth Control Pills

I have already discussed the likelihood hormones play a role in SOD. There are quite a few women who claim their SOD goes away when they are on birth control and cannot go off it without having severe SOD symptoms return. There are also women who developed SOD symptoms by going on birth control or hormone replacement therapy. There is very little consistency or predictability when it comes to hormone therapy and its effects on SOD symptoms. Birth control having a positive effect would make sense because the same holds true for most women who are pregnant, a time when progesterone and estrogen are high.

Birth control that seems to be the most effective for helping SOD symptoms is one that is a low dose of both estrogen and progesterone. Women whose birth control is only a progesterone or who take estrogen hormone replacement therapy seem to do worse. Possibly having too much of one hormone creates an unfavorable balance and it somehow affects the sphincter of Oddi. This isn't always the case, though. Some women who have been diagnosed "estrogen dominant" claim remission of their SOD symptoms taking a progesterone-only pill or applying a progesterone cream.

The low dose birth control I am on definitely helps my right side pain. Unfortunately, I have to take periodic breaks from taking it. Birth control can cause dangerous side effects like blood clots and strokes particularly in middle age women like me.

Medication Safety and Side Effects

I was the type of person who relied on pills to cure whatever ailed me. Had a headache? Took a pill. Felt sad? Went to the doctor to get a pill. Had a slight infection? Hurry up and get an antibiotic. Now I run far away from a prescription pad unless I know a medicine will save my life or greatly improve my quality of life and not disable or kill me in the process. This change in attitude came at a cost after I had a severe long term adverse reaction to a fluoroquinolone antibiotic. (think Cipro, Avelox, Levaquin, etc.). This reaction has left me with severe neuropathy, connective tissue problems, and a completely messed up central nervous system.

As of this writing, it has been three and a half years since I was given the antibiotic and many of my symptoms appear to be permanent. I never thought an antibiotic could do so much damage but it did. Now there are black box warnings from the FDA about these drugs, not that I would have paid attention. I never thought severe side effects would happen to me. No, that happens to other people.

This adverse reaction also triggered an inability to tolerate most medications. If there is a rare side effect, I get it. Some with this same adverse reaction attribute this to a corrupted liver enzyme system. Most medications are metabolized in the liver where this organ's enzymes and detoxification pathways are responsible for converting medication to its active component and removing its associated toxins from the body.

Ideally, this process runs smoothly with few problems. This is not the case for all people or medications. Genetic mutations can play a major role in how you tolerate a particular medication. I found out an incredible amount of information relative to my genetics by consulting with a natural health practitioner specializing in epigenetics/genomics. She had me order DNA testing through www.23andme.com, then went over my genetic mutations and recommended a supplement, diet, and lifestyle plan for my genetic body type. She also explained why I struggled with some medications.

My reason for mentioning all of this isn't to scare you completely away from medications, but to encourage you to be cautious with any prescription or over the counter medication you consider taking for SOD. Ask your doctor if there are black box warnings for a medication and what the most common side effects are for any drug. Get to know your pharmacist and let him or her know you want to be alerted of possible drug interactions and severe side effects.

Also, ask your pharmacist to alert you if "spasm of sphincter of Oddi" is a side effect of any drug you are prescribed. I just discovered a few days ago that a side effect of acetaminophen is spasm of sphincter of Oddi. I thought the only medications I needed to worry about were opioid pain medications. Not the case.

Remember, doctors and pharmacists don't always know every side effect and many aren't listed in the product's post marketing materials. I can't tell you how many times a doctor or pharmacist told me a strange symptom I was experiencing could not be from the drug I was taking. Consequently, I would cease taking the drug and the side effect would go away or improve. Always go with your gut instinct. There is a reason .0001% of people get a side effect and the rest of the population don't. Everyone is unique and thanks to our genetics we metabolize drugs differently.

Chapter 9: Procedural and Surgical Treatments

When all else fails, and SOD symptoms are not improved with diet, medications or natural healing methods, more invasive measures may need to be considered. Going the invasive procedural or surgical route is not a decision to be taken lightly. I have witnessed quite a few SOD patients, including myself, come close to dying from acute pancreatitis, sepsis infections and other complications of procedures and surgeries. Regardless, in some cases, procedures or surgeries are the only options for an SOD patient to have a quality and seemingly normal life.

Arriving at the decision to have an invasive procedure or surgery is one that is usually born out of desperation. You would do just about anything to feel better, including risk your life. Some SOD sufferers have such severe symptoms it is impossible for them to live a normal life. This can cause anyone to make a drastic, potentially life changing decision, with the hope of getting better. However, just as I have witnessed the ill effects of invasive treatments, I have witnessed many success stories. Therefore, it is impossible to know who will benefit from which procedure. Please consider the following when deciding on a procedure or surgery:

What are the statistical chances this procedure/surgery will work?
What risks are associated with the procedure/surgery?
Do the risks outweigh the possible benefits?
How long will it take to recover from the procedure/surgery?
How will my pain be managed after the procedure/surgery?

If you are considering an invasive procedure I strongly suggest you join an online SOD support group or forum to find out how others faired with that same procedure. Each person is different but it may help you to make an informed decision. It will also give you a snapshot of best and worst case scenarios. It may frighten you to hear a story of a near death experience with a procedure you already have scheduled. But it may force you to reconsider whether you really need the procedure and learn about precautions to consider if you go through with the procedure.

If you are determined to have an invasive procedure, you can also learn from others of what is a realistic recovery period. Doctors will give you an estimated number of days you will be hospitalized or insist a procedure will be outpatient. I know I am a rare exception and a "Murphy" but both times I had invasive procedures I needed to stay in the hospital way longer than expected.

My ERCP was supposed to be outpatient and turned into a week-long hospital stay including four days in an intensive care unit. My transduodenal sphincteroplasty surgery was supposed to be a week-long hospital stay but ended up being a month. I am a rare exception. The majority of SOD patients who have procedures and surgeries don't experience this but, again, be informed.

I may come across as seeming to be "anti-procedure" or "anti-surgery" but I am not. This book is written as a survival guide and as such it would be irresponsible of me to not inform the reader of both the good and the bad aspects of invasive treatments.

I have compiled a list of the most common procedures and surgeries performed for treating SOD. I did not include cholecystectomy (gallbladder removal) as it often triggers SOD or makes SOD worse. I personally would not have a cholecystectomy to treat SOD. But, I do know a select few who had terrible SOD symptoms and a cholecystectomy pretty much cured them. Those stories are few in comparison to the number of SOD sufferers whose symptoms developed or worsened following cholecystectomy.

Obviously, if you have a diseased gallbladder get it removed. But if there is no good reason to remove it I would keep mine. I also don't include information about surgeries meant to primarily treat chronic pancreatitis and other pancreatic conditions like the Whipple, Frey, or Total Pancreatectomy with Auto Islet Transfer (TP-AIT).

Botox

Botulinum toxin (Botox), a potent inhibitor of acetylcholine release from nerve endings, is injected during an endoscopy procedure. About 50% of SOD patients experience symptom relief from this procedure as it reduces basal sphincter pressure. Think of it this way. If a woman gets Botox in her forehead, it freezes the muscles so she doesn't have any forehead lines. I'll confess I had Botox a few times, several years ago. It was miraculous, but I didn't like how I couldn't raise my eyebrows. Same goes for Botox in the sphincter. It freezes the sphincter, preventing it from spasm.

This reduction in pressure may be accompanied by symptom improvement in some patients. For some, Botox is a promising alternative to more invasive procedures. The risks of complications are fewer than with most other invasive procedures. The patient is sedated and the endoscopy tube sent down the esophagus to the duodenum. There, the Botox is applied.

When risks do arise they are likely to be associated with either the anesthesia or the Botox itself as an allergy or sensitivity. Other than that there could be minor side effects related to the placement of the endoscopy tube. Though this is one of the safest procedures, the downfall is Botox wears off within a few months and must be repeated, generally, at a minimum of every six months. Overall, the majority of SOD patients who respond to botulinum toxin versus those who didn't gain any pain relief later benefited from endoscopic sphincterotomy. Therefore, Botox is a good indicator of whether sphincterotomy will work.

Few physicians perform Botox injections for SOD, at least in the United States. I don't know why this is. Maybe it is a health insurance issue? It doesn't make sense if something can bring relief without deadly side effects. Why not make it available to all? As of this writing, there is a doctor in New York who started using Botox. I believe a doctor in Florida performs it as well. I am unaware of others. I know of a male SOD patient in the United Kingdom who gets regular Botox injections for his SOD. He has it done several times a year and is able to have a quality of life thanks to this procedure.

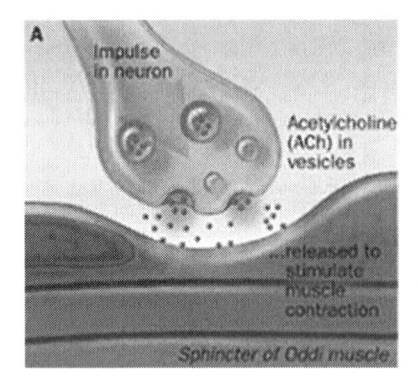

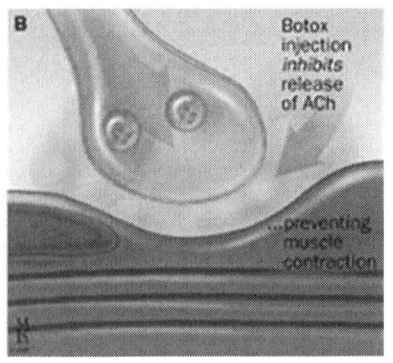

Celiac Plexus Block

A celiac plexus block is an injection of local anesthetic into or around the celiac plexus of nerves that surrounds the aorta, the main artery in the abdomen. These nerves can carry pain information from the gut or abdominal organ tissues back to the spinal cord and brain. It can be injected into the abdomen, back, or via EUS. On occasion, in addition to a local anesthetic, epinephrine, clonidine or a steroid medication may be added to prolong the effects of the celiac plexus block. In extreme cases, the doctor will inject alcohol which will kill the nerve.

I had a celiac plexus block performed through the abdomen last year for my pancreatic pain. I never had it done when I had SOD pain. The procedure did absolutely nothing for the pain. However, I know several SOD patients who had it performed via EUS and had SOD pain relief for several months. Usually, an anesthesiologist or gastroenterologist will perform this as an outpatient procedure. Most patients receive sedation so the patient doesn't feel the needle and injection. There is a risk of infection, bleeding, collapsed lung, arterial puncture, nerve damage or drug allergy. There can also be a reaction from the injected medication or from IV sedation or very rarely paralysis. Most commonly the patient may develop low blood pressure or diarrhea.

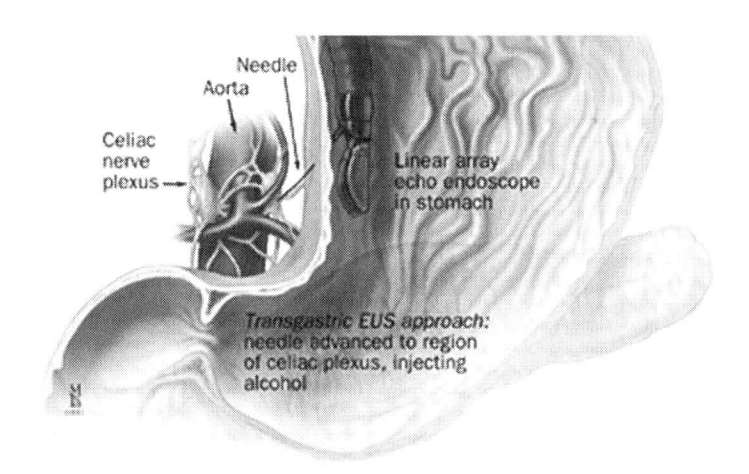

Figure labels: Celiac nerve plexus, Aorta, Needle, Linear array echo endoscope in stomach, Transgastric EUS approach: needle advanced to region of celiac plexus, injecting alcohol

Spinal Cord Stimulator

A spinal cord stimulator is a medical device surgically implanted under your skin that sends a mild electric current to your spinal cord. A small wire carries the current from a pulse generator to the nerve fibers of the spinal cord. When turned on, the stimulation feels like a mild tingling in the area where the pain is felt. Your pain is reduced because the electrical current interrupts the pain signal from reaching your brain. Stimulation does not eliminate the source of pain, it simply interferes with the signal to the brain, and so the amount of pain relief varies for each person.

A trial period and psychological evaluation are also required to ensure the patient can handle the responsibility of an implantable device, will achieve pain relief, and the stimulation is not unpleasant. The goal for spinal cord stimulation is a 50-70% reduction in pain. Many pain management doctors are pushing their patients to get stimulators. It absolutely could benefit SOD patients but know that stimulation does not work for everyone and there are serious risks to consider, including paralysis.

Also, the body could form adhesions around the device, which may prevent it from ever being removed. I know firsthand two individuals who experienced this. Unfortunately, the device lost its efficacy and then because of adhesions will remain in their bodies for a lifetime. Other risks include infection, bleeding, headache, allergic reaction, spinal fluid leakage, paralysis, and issues specific to the spinal cord stimulator and lead wires. If your pain is severely affecting your life this may be the last resort solution, especially if doctors are completely resistant to prescribing pain medication.

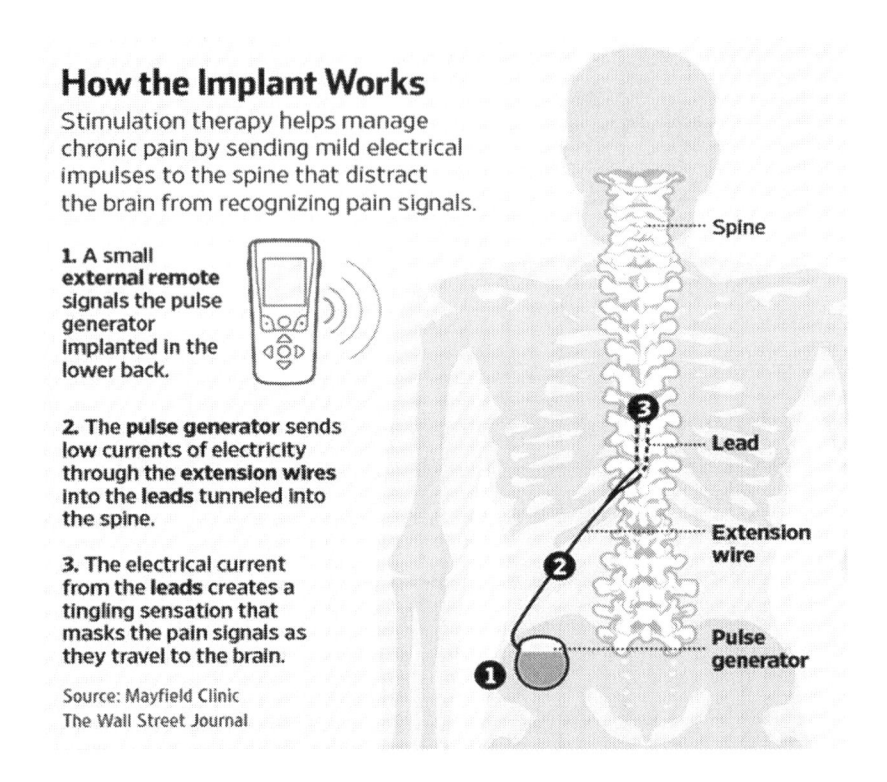

How the Implant Works

Stimulation therapy helps manage chronic pain by sending mild electrical impulses to the spine that distract the brain from recognizing pain signals.

1. A small **external remote** signals the pulse generator implanted in the lower back.

2. The **pulse generator** sends low currents of electricity through the **extension wires** into the **leads** tunneled into the spine.

3. The electrical current from the **leads** creates a tingling sensation that masks the pain signals as they travel to the brain.

Source: Mayfield Clinic
The Wall Street Journal

Stent Placement

Stents are placed into the bile or pancreatic duct to bypass strictures, or narrowed parts of the duct, and to help keep the sphincters wide and open. There are two types of stents that are commonly used. The first is made of plastic and looks like a small straw. A plastic stent can be pushed through the ERCP scope into a blocked duct to allow normal drainage. The second type of stent is made of metal wires that look like the cross wires of a fence or cage. The metal stent is flexible, expandable and springs open to a larger diameter than plastic stents.

Both plastic and metal stents tend to clog up after several months and may require another ERCP to swap out for a new stent. Metal stents are more permanent while plastic stents are easily removed at a repeat procedure. Your doctor will choose the best type of stent for your problem. Something I noticed in support groups was the SOD patients who benefited from biliary stents did not benefit as much from sphincterotomy or sphincteroplasty. They did, however, benefit greatly from biliary roux en y surgeries. This is important to note if you are considering a sphincteroplasty or a biliary roux en y. I know a few SOD patients who went through major sphincteroplasty surgery only to then have a biliary roux en y surgery.

Pancreatic stents can help with SOD and chronic pancreatitis symptoms but their insertion may disturb the temperamental and sensitive pancreas. Stents are not ever meant to be permanent. And though it may be a bother to get them routinely swapped out, it may be worth the hassle to avoid the risks of other more invasive solutions. The risks of stent placement include acute pancreatitis (from pancreatic stent placement), ductal perforation, and any risks involved with anesthesia and endoscopy.

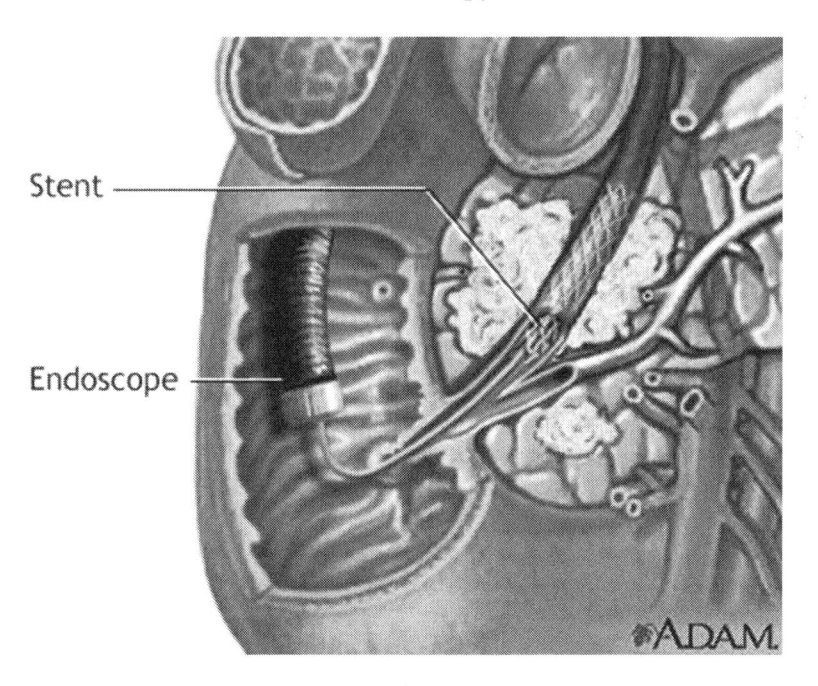

Balloon Dilation/Dilatation

During an ERCP, a physician will use a catheter fitted with a dilating balloon to stretch the sphincter and duct area. This balloon is inflated with a sterile saline solution up to a size (at least > 10 mm in diameter) and duration (usually 2–6 min) according to the patients' condition and tolerance. The balloon is then inflated to stretch out the narrowing. In order to minimize the risk of perforation, the size of the balloon should not exceed the size of the common bile duct. This procedure is often used to remove stones lodged in the bile duct. It is also used to sweep out biliary sludge and debris.

Dilation with balloons is often performed when the cause of the narrowing is benign (not cancer). After balloon dilation, a temporary stent may be placed for a few months to help maintain the dilation. Risks are the same for balloon dilatation as they are for stents. Also, the balloon could break and get stuck in the duct, which will of course need retrieval.

Sphincterotomy

Sphincterotomy is cutting of the sphincter muscle. It is generally an outpatient procedure in which you will prepare as you would for an endoscopy and be sedated. The cut is made to enlarge the opening while your doctor looks through the ERCP scope at the papilla or duct opening. A small wire on a specialized catheter uses electric current to cut the tissue. The actual cut is quite small, usually less than 1/2 inch. This small cut also allows various treatments in the ducts, like stent placement and sweeping of the ducts.

Two cuts can be made. The most common is to the entrance of the bile duct, called a biliary sphincterotomy. Sometimes that is enough to bring relief for the SOD patient. Alternatively, if the biliary sphincterotomy alone does not help and it is suspected or proven the pancreatic sphincter has high pressures, a cut will be made in both the biliary sphincter and pancreatic sphincter.

When nothing solved my SOD symptoms I begged for a sphincterotomy. My local doctors refused to do an ERCP let alone a sphincterotomy. I was desperate and furious. I flew across the country and finally had it done. I had the "full Monty" so to speak—ERCP with manometry, dual sphincterotomy and stents placed in my bile and pancreatic ducts. I was very ill afterward but had some relief of symptoms for about a month before I reverted back to all the same disabling symptoms, hence the reason I went forward with major surgery. Though I had a less than successful experience, the majority of people I know with SOD benefit from this procedure.

Deciding on whether to have a sphincterotomy may come down to what SOD Type you are. Based on research, the Hogan-Geenen sphincter of Oddi classification described statistically the likelihood patients would achieve pain relief from sphincterotomy, depending on their SOD Type. Type 1 patients have the highest success rate for pain relief post-sphincterotomy at about 90-95%. Type 2 patients have less favorable results at 35-85% depending on whether their manometry was normal or abnormal.

The recent Evaluating Predictors and Interventions in Sphincter of Oddi Dysfunction (EPISOD) study showed that Type 3 patients did not benefit any better than the placebo group for sphincterotomy. That is not to say no SOD Type 3 patient benefited from sphincterotomy. They just did about the same as the placebo group. The Hogan-Geenen classification concluded symptom relief was achieved by 55-65% of SOD Type 3 patients after sphincterotomy if they had abnormal manometry. If their manometry was normal, the success rate was less than 10%.

The most common and serious risk of ERCP is acute pancreatitis. This can occur in up to 30% of the population and is three times more likely to happen if the person is suspected of having SOD as opposed to the general population. Another risk factor is SOD patients with Type 3 are more likely to develop acute pancreatitis following an ERCP. Performing a manometry has not shown to be an added risk factor for acute pancreatitis. Placement of a prophylactic pancreatic duct stent has been shown to limit the incidence of acute pancreatitis as has pre-procedural administration of an indomethacin (NSAID) suppository. If you decide to have an ERCP with sphincterotomy, be sure to ask your doctor if he can include them in your procedure.

Other risks with sphincterotomy are bleeding (always tell your doctor what medications you are on, especially those that may interfere with blood clotting), ductal injury, infection, and anything that may arise as a risk factor with anesthesia and an endoscopy. A somewhat benign side effect of sphincterotomy but worth mentioning is reflux of duodenal contents. This happens because the opening is wider and the sphincter sometimes stays open once it is cut. Rarely, duodenal reflux contents can accumulate in the duct and cause a blockage. Sphincterotomy commonly needs to be repeated as stenosis and scar tissue/adhesions can develop in the sphincter area. Stenosis occurs when, over time, the area heals tighter and tighter.

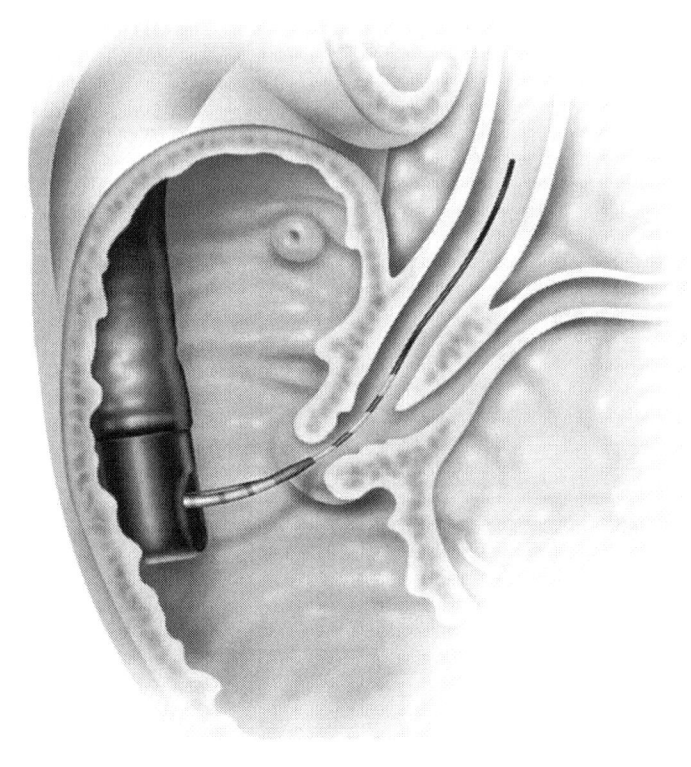

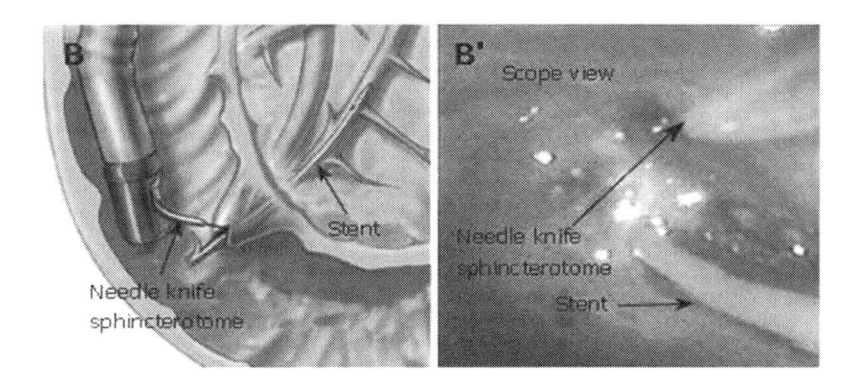

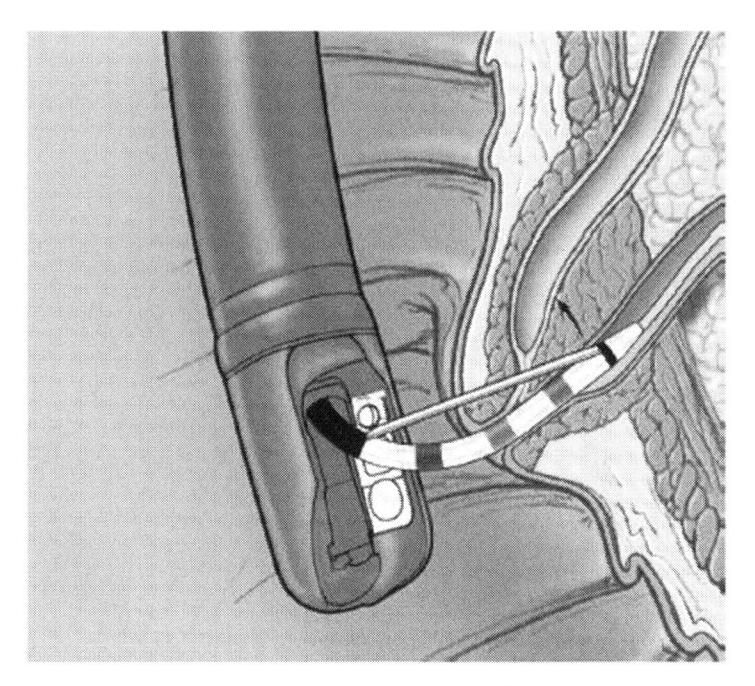

Figure 7 Transpancreatic precut sphincterotomy

Transduodenal Sphincteroplasty

Transduodenal means "through the duodenum." When a doctor performs a sphincteroplasty he or she slices and sews the sphincter permanently open. Gastroenterologists generally do not perform this type of surgery. A surgeon specializing in biliary and pancreatic surgery may perform it as a laparotomy or laparoscopic surgery. A laparotomy is a surgical procedure involving a large incision through the abdominal wall to gain access into the abdominal cavity.

Laparotomy requires a very long recovery period as several layers of skin and muscle are cut. Laparoscopic surgery is a technique in which an operation is conducted using small incisions and a laparoscope. The laparoscope has a camera so the surgeon can see clearly the area he must operate since it is beneath the skin, muscle, and possibly other organs. Many complex laparoscopic surgeries today use a robot to make incisions and access areas a surgeon's hands cannot.

There are a number of advantages to laparoscopic surgery versus laparotomy. Pain and bleeding are reduced due to smaller incisions and recovery times often shorter. Unfortunately, as of this writing, very few surgeons perform this surgery laparoscopically. I had this surgery as a laparotomy and it took at least three to four months before I could perform gentle exercises. I will not lie. It was incredibly painful—so painful they had me on a ketamine (a horse tranquilizer) and oxymorphone (Dilaudid) IV drip for the pain. I ended up with a sepsis infection and nearly died. I remained in the hospital a month.

Also, the sphincteroplasty opened the floodgates of bile. It was gushing for a few weeks after the surgery. I had a drain that filled constantly. I also had excessive bile diarrhea to the point I had to be on IV fluids constantly. The typical sphincteroplasty hospital stay is a week. Again, I am a Murphy and an extreme case. All other SOD patients I know who had a sphincteroplasty were out of the hospital within a week and did well, for the most part.

The sphincteroplasty doesn't seem to "cure" anyone's SOD entirely, at least no one I have met. There is not much in the way of research measuring the success of sphincteroplasty in SOD patients. However, a 1985 study in the *Annals of Surgery* showed 77%

of transduodenal sphincteroplasty patients achieved excellent or good results for a variety of disorders and conditions. Many SOD patients who had a sphincteroplasty, including me, end up with chronic pancreatitis.

It is unclear why, but possibly it could be from the free reflux of duodenal contents into the ducts now that this area is completely wide open all of the time. Possibly those of us who had acute pancreatitis from an ERCP were bound to develop chronic pancreatitis eventually. Theories abound and so much is unknown. For some, continuing problems and chronic pancreatitis are caused by a "re-stenosis" of the sphincter area and/or accumulation of scar tissue, i.e. adhesions.

I apologize this all sounds so doom and gloom. It may sound hard to believe, but though I had a terrible time after the surgery, I do not regret having had the sphincteroplasty. Prior to the surgery, I was very ill and absolutely nothing else was helping. A few months after the surgery I gained back the weight I desperately needed, my right side SOD pain diminished, and my 24/7 nausea was gone. The other SOD patients I know who had this surgery had similar results. I still had some right side pain but it was manageable. Transduodenal sphincteroplasty risks include bleeding, infection, and common surgical complications. Rarely will a sphincteroplasty cause acute pancreatitis.

Transduodenal Sphincteroplasty

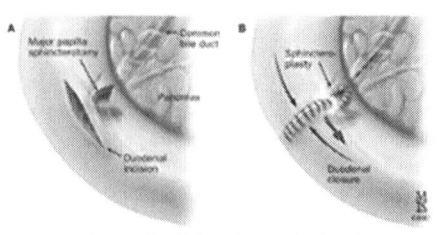

Above: Incision through duodenum

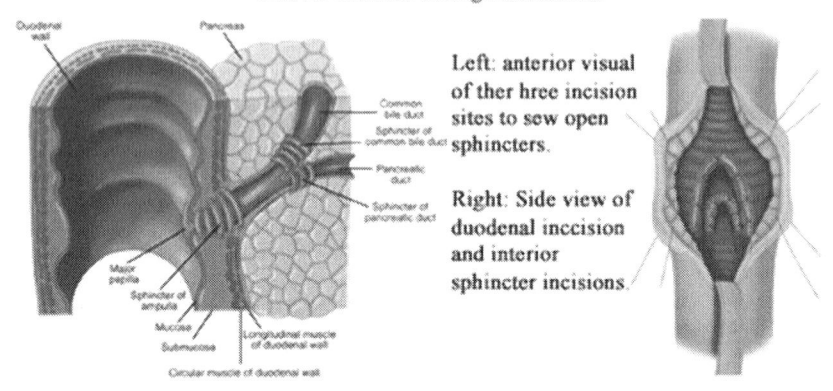

Left: anterior visual of ther hree incision sites to sew open sphincters.

Right: Side view of duodenal inccision and interior sphincter incisions.

Biliary Roux En Y

Biliary roux en y surgery is the nickname for any surgery involving an anastomosis (cutting then reconnecting) of the common bile duct to the duodenum or another cut portion of the small intestine (known as the roux en y limb), diverting it away from the stomach and pancreas. Choledochojejunostomy seems to be the procedure of choice for SOD surgeons performing a biliary roux en y. Other biliary roux en y surgeries are the hepaticojejunostomy and choledochoduodenostomy. Traditionally, biliary roux en y surgery is indicated for patients with recurrent gallstones requiring repeated intervention, impacted or giant stones, biliary sludge, ampullary stenosis, diseased or cancerous bile duct, dilated lower common bile duct, and restoring continuity to the biliary tract.

For SOD patients, the bile duct and small intestine are cut and then sewn together over by the liver. The patient's stomach contents (chyme) and pancreatic enzymes continue to empty into the duodenum. But now as this is happening the liver is emptying bile through the bile duct into another area of the small intestine, not the duodenum. The bile will eventually meet up with the chyme and pancreatic enzymes.

So how will this help the SOD patient? First, the biliary sphincter is in a sense obliterated when the anatomy is restructured. Every SOD patient I know who had biliary SOD issues, especially those who acquired relief from stents, appeared "cured" after having a biliary roux en y. Pain and nausea became non-existent or drastically reduced. If someone had pancreatic issues, these individuals continued to have trouble with their pancreas and pancreatic duct like those who had the sphincteroplasty.

Biliary roux en y is major surgery that can be done as a laparotomy or laparoscopically. This particular surgery can cause repeated episodes of cholangitis—a bacterial infection in the bile duct because of translocated bacteria migrating upwards to the jejunal portion of the small intestine, into the bile duct and liver. Other possible complications are hemorrhaging, bile leaks, strictures (narrowing of the bile duct) and any surgery-related complications.

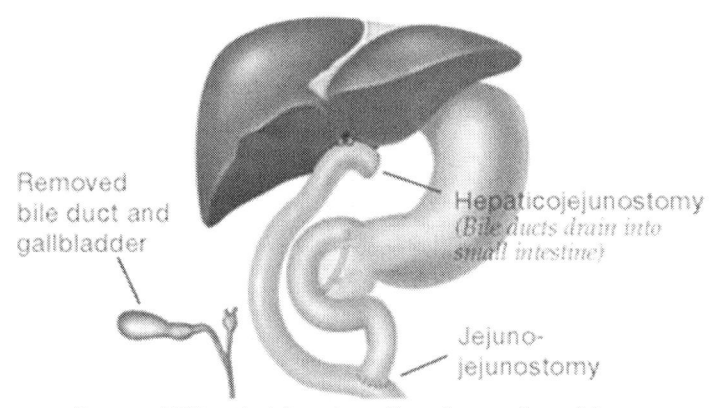

Roux-en-Y Hepaticojejunostomy Procedure performed for cholangiocarcinoma and biliary injuries.

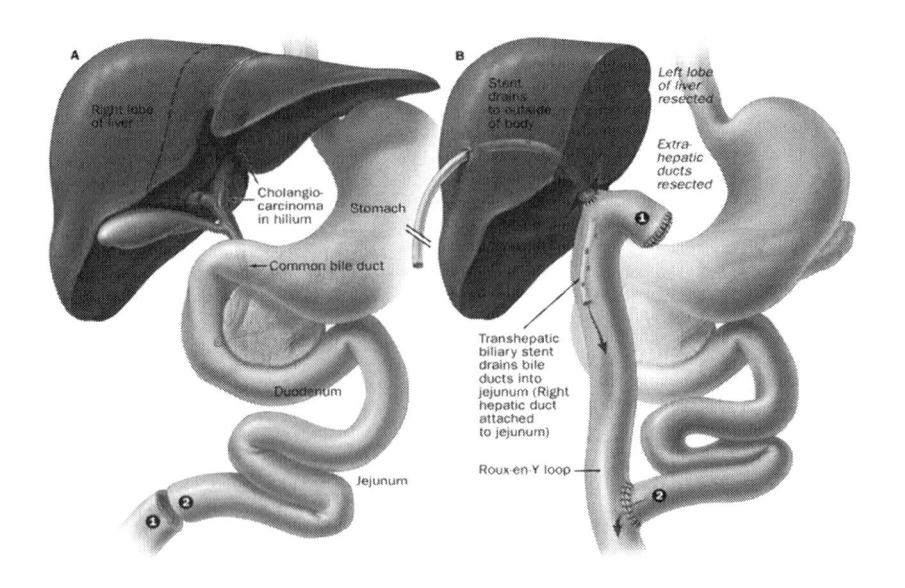

Feeding Tubes

I was conflicted about where to include information about feeding tubes. Since the majority of feeding tubes require a surgical procedure to place them, I figured this was the right chapter. Feeding tubes won't cure SOD but they can aid in reducing symptoms and provide nourishment in extreme cases. The most common feeding tubes for SOD patients are the gastrostomy-jejunostomy (G/J)—through the stomach and small intestine—and jejunostomy (J)—only through the small intestine—tubes. There is also the nasogastric tube which enters through the nose but is usually reserved for temporary tube feedings like in a hospital setting. Both the G/J and J tubes deliver nutrient-rich liquid formula to the jejunal section of the small intestine. This bypasses the sphincter area and theoretically will not trigger the sphincter or pancreas. This, of course, doesn't always happen. All digestive organs can be stimulated instinctually once food enters any part of the body.

I had both of these types of feeding tubes at different times. They were fraught with complications from the beginning. The first time

I had one placed, the pain from the surgical placement was pretty bad so I stayed in the hospital a few days. The second time wasn't terrible. The tube kept migrating and formula would backwash up passed the sphincter area and into the stomach, defeating the purpose of the feeding tube. Another time the tube kinked and I couldn't get the formula to flow. It also took over a month to get the formula right. Add to all this the nuisance of having to hook up to the machine several times a day. Regardless though I had many complications from my feeding tubes and the formula, they certainly served their purpose in helping me gain weight.

After my sphincteroplasty I had a peripherally inserted central catheter (PICC) line that delivered total parenteral nutrition (TPN). The PICC line is a central line placed into a large vein usually in the upper arm where liquid nutrition is slowly delivered to the body intravenously. I usually ran it at night to give me freedom during the day. It wasn't so bad but easily got infected and I had to be super careful to not get the lines wet.

I don't know a single person who didn't have issues with feeding tubes and PICC lines. All of them are susceptible to infections, line complications, and can dislodge. However, if you are losing weight at a dangerous rate and can't eat much, one of these alternative nutrition sources may be necessary. I know very few SOD patients who needed a feeding tube or PICC line permanently. Most SOD patients go through short periods of needing them, then bounce back and do fine without them. Those who needed them permanently had a comorbidity disease like gastroparesis, chronic pancreatitis, and Ehlers-Danlos Syndrome.

G-J or J-tubes are usually inserted/placed by a surgeon. PICC lines can be placed by an interventional radiologist. Dieticians, primary care doctors, gastroenterologists, surgeons, and nutritional medical doctors can all manage feeding tube formula and TPN prescriptions. Typically, you will need a visiting nurse come to your home to help you get started with your feeds and monitor your progress. These services are almost always covered by health insurance. The visiting nurse assigned to me was a doll. I looked forward to her weekly visits and was actually depressed when I knew I didn't need the feeding tubes anymore as I missed her company.

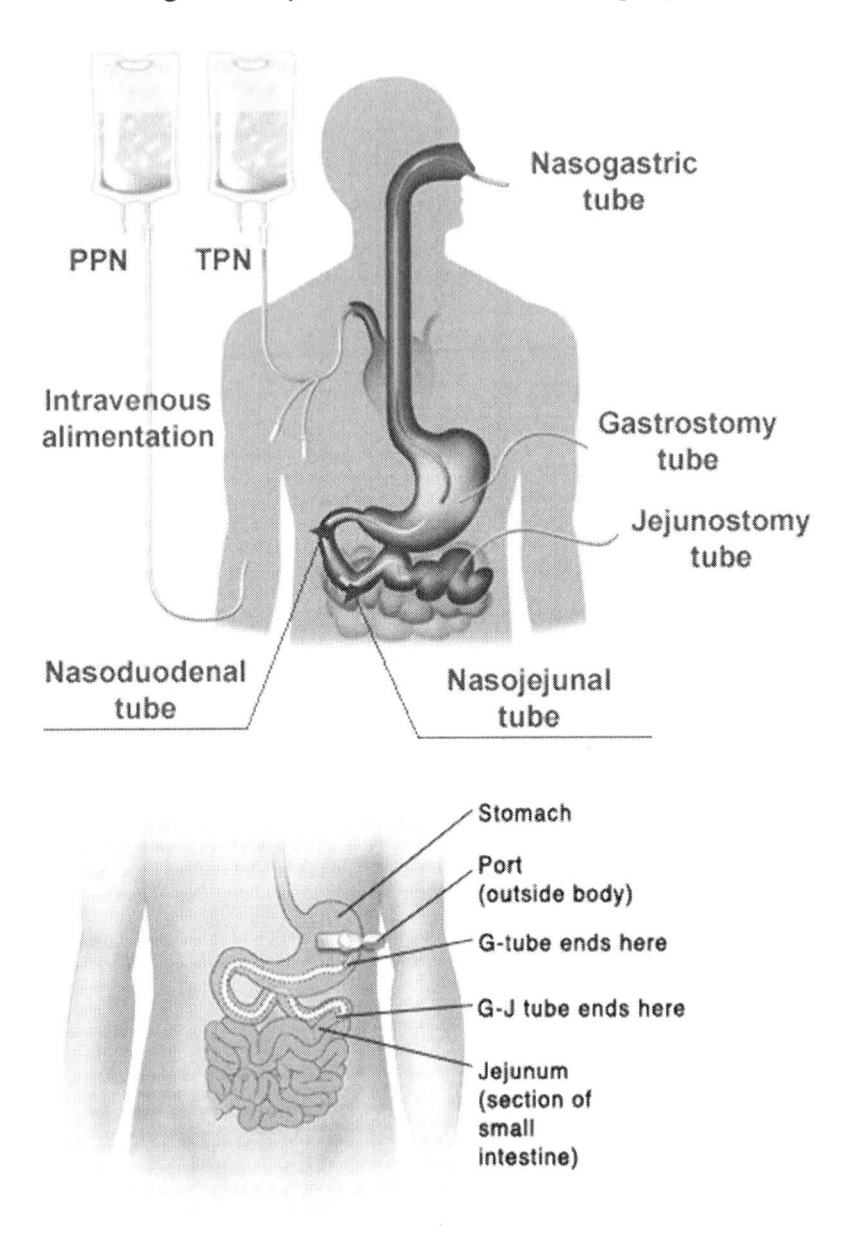

PPN TPN

Nasogastric tube

Intravenous alimentation

Gastrostomy tube

Jejunostomy tube

Nasoduodenal tube

Nasojejunal tube

Stomach
Port (outside body)
G-tube ends here
G-J tube ends here
Jejunum (section of small intestine)

Chapter 10: Self-Care and Support

You have been through rounds of testing, been jabbed so many times with IV needles you feel like a human pin cushion. You are relieved you have a name to your condition but your symptoms still plague you. Possibly you have minor symptoms and have had success utilizing a more natural treatment approach. Or, you may be in remission and are waiting for the proverbial shoe to drop. Whatever has brought you here or keeps you here, or how severe or benign your SOD symptoms are, it is important you take measures to take care of yourself.

How do you go about taking care of yourself? The most important thing is to find your own tried and true self-care tools and put them in an imaginary self-care toolbox. This way you will know what to try when things go awry. We are all different and what one person may like or need can be vastly different from the next person. I like to get facials, pedicures and massages while someone else may hate to be touched. I also love yoga and hiking, while another person with SOD may like to jog, something I have never liked doing.

My first suggestion is to re-read Chapter 6: Natural Treatments again and use it as a reference for ideas on how to naturally keep symptoms at bay. Many of the natural treatments suggested can be used to achieve emotional balance as well and aid with other physical conditions related to your SOD or not. Guided meditations and yoga can be used to de-stress and achieve emotional wellness. They aren't solely for managing SOD pain. There are literally hundreds of ways you can be kind to yourself and self-soothe.

Support groups

Support groups can be both helpful or make matters worse. Many people who frequent SOD support groups are in the throes of illness and pain. Keep in mind when people experience remission or freedom from SOD symptoms the last place they will likely be is in a support group. Instead, they will be out living their lives and making up for lost time from when they were ill. A few of us stick around to give back and offer support and hope but we are few and far between. It is unfortunate when people who are doing well leave support groups as it can seem dismal and hopeless if you are in a support group with no healthy people.

I had a friend with mysterious symptoms similar to SOD join my SOD group. I thought it would help her get support so she didn't feel so alone with her symptoms. Well, she ended up fleeing the group just as soon as I added her. The stories of people suffering and the length of time they suffered was frightening. She is doing well today and ended up benefiting from natural treatments. I completely understood and it got me to thinking how unfortunate it is that so many people don't stick around to show people there is hope and to just hang in there. Support groups are not for everyone.

I had the opposite experience with support groups. When I found my first SOD support group I was relieved. I was no longer alone. I met others who had the same symptoms and often the exact same experiences with the health care system, unless they received care in Minnesota or Indiana (I rarely heard bad reports from these folks). I had gone several months feeling like I was the only person on the planet with my illness. The support group was helpful because at that time I was not yet officially diagnosed with SOD. I was able to get information that did not exist anywhere on the Internet or from the mouths of any of my doctors. I no longer doubted myself because my doctors refused to consider SOD as a diagnosis.

Worse, my local doctors consistently treated me as though my symptoms were all in my head. I was starting to wonder if I was indeed losing my mind and there would be no end in sight, no diagnosis or treatment. For me, it was reassuring to meet others with the same experiences—good and bad. It also gave me the opportunity to learn from others. In an online support forum, I found the name of the doctor who ultimately diagnosed me. I learned about natural treatments that helped others. I got support with my nightmare feeding tube when I was at a loss of what to do.

Over the past four years since joining my first SOD support group, I have witnessed just about every possible SOD scenario and been through so much that I could relate to nearly every support group member's post. I probably would have never written this book if I never found an SOD support group. I certainly would not have gathered half the information I wrote in this book as I learned much of it at one time or another from other SOD patients.

You can find support groups on Facebook by putting in the keywords "SOD" or "Sphincter of Oddi Dysfunction" in the search field at the top. Groups will appear as suggested pages or groups. Most are the same but with different rules, moderators, and number of group members. The Facebook support group I run is at https://www.facebook.com/groups/SODAE/. Other support groups can be found online by searching Internet search engines like Google, Yahoo! or Bing. The website Inspire.com has several digestive disease-specific groups. I have never heard of anyone running a face to face SOD support group or an online chat or video group. Maybe someone will start one someday.

If anonymity is a major issue for you, I recommend using a friend's or family member's online account or make up a pseudonym for an online account. You don't have to participate in online support groups to benefit from them. You can simply lurk and read others' posts. I used the search tool in the Facebook groups to find specific things I wanted to know when I didn't want to post. Usually, this field is at the top right or somewhere you can put in a keyword and search through posts. For example, say you are too embarrassed to ask about bile diarrhea. Instead of posting, you can search in the group's search field for "bile diarrhea." The searches generally go back several years so you should see everything anyone ever wrote about bile diarrhea.

Be cautious with online support groups as not everyone is there for the same reason and some aren't even really sick. Yes, there are actually people faking disease. I caught a woman blatantly lying about her condition and copying verbatim someone else's story. Be careful who you befriend. I only converse with people who have real names and profile photos. After a while, you can discern who is real and who may not be who they say they are.

I do have support group friends who I've engaged in phone conversations. There is even a group of us who send holiday greeting cards to each other. Some support group members have gotten me through the worst days—as much as my family or "well" friends because they could relate. Having something in common, even a bad thing like SOD is therapeutic. I feel safe with my online friends and know they have my back whenever I need them. Some are like sisters to me.

My friend Kelly has been the greatest blessing. She somehow found me on a support group forum and sent me an email asking about my experience with the pancreatic enzyme, Creon. I don't know how it all happened but we became the best of friends. Though much of our friendship has been via email and she lives on the west coast while I live on the east coast, we make a point to meet up in New York City once a year and now talk on the phone and text nearly every day. She has been my biggest supporter and cheerleader. It is amazing the blessings that can come out of something so awful.

Mental Health Therapy

If you search the Internet for "mental health therapy for cancer patients," thousands of search results appear, including anything from where to get therapy to resources for support groups, general information, research on the mental effects of cancer, etc. The American Cancer Society has online modules for patients on how to mentally and emotionally deal with anything related to their illness. It was really no surprise that when I conducted the same type of search for SOD, I found nothing except a few research articles stating anxiety and depression could cause SOD or those with SOD may have higher instances of anxiety and depression.

I can attest that many patients with SOD, like those with cancer, experience debilitating anxiety and depression symptoms, a direct result of their illness and everything that goes along with it. From my experience, it is also common for SOD patients to develop a form of health-related post-traumatic stress disorder (PTSD). Many of them complain they developed a fear of doctors and hospitals, a fear of eating, and a fear of illness in general. Some avoid doing things they used to enjoy for fear it will cause an SOD flare up. Poor mental health status has been known to exacerbate health conditions and contribute to poor health outcomes.

By the time I recuperated from my health crisis, I had developed an intense fear and resentment of doctors and hospitals. I have had many severe pancreatic pain episodes over the past year yet I refused to go to the emergency room because of my health-related PTSD. There are many contributing factors to my PTSD, including mistreatment by health care staff and doctors, doctors not believing me, being treated as a drug seeker because of normal test results, isolation from society, nearly dying, spending a good portion of a year in the hospital, and just the fact I was sick 24/7 for several years.

The best thing I did for my emotional and mental well-being was sought help from a qualified mental health therapist. Therapists who focus on trauma issues are ideal for SOD patients. A therapist once told me that the form of PTSD I had from my health nightmare was akin to those coming back from war or patients who survived stage 4 cancer. I say that not to downplay the severity of those types of PTSD. Instead, never underestimate the damage this condition can do to one's mental, emotional, and spiritual state.

If you have had perfect care from doctors and healthcare staff, and minimal symptoms then maybe you cannot relate to how bad it could possibly be. If this is the case, kudos to you and count yourself very fortunate. I have met many SOD patients who get diagnosed immediately, have access to any and all SOD treatments, and have compassionate doctors. Their SOD has very little effect on their mental state. They cannot understand how horrible it is for those of us fighting for care. What I went through and the majority of others go through is beyond traumatic. It is horrible and beyond tortuous. Some have taken their lives because of this disease and lack of proper healthcare.

The best form of therapy I received was from the hypnotherapist I saw for pain. He helped teach me coping and self-soothing skills not only for my pain but also for the mental anguish I endured, which was a whole other type of pain. He also incorporated evidenced-based trauma treatment techniques. I also saw a few therapists before him who were helpful but the therapies seemed to run their course and I needed to move on.

There are many different types of therapy. I personally only see therapists trained in at least one evidence-based modality. Some of the most common therapies for trauma are Cognitive Behavioral Therapy (CBT), Narrative Exposure, Prolonged Exposure, and Eye Movement Desensitization and Reprocessing (EMDR). Most psychotherapists are versed in CBT or "Talk Therapy.

I had positive results with CBT, which focuses on exploring relationships among a person's thoughts, feelings, and behaviors. During CBT a therapist will actively work with a person to uncover unhealthy patterns of thought and how they may be causing self-destructive behaviors and beliefs. CBT helps you become aware of inaccurate or negative thinking so you can view challenging situations more clearly and respond to them in a more effective way.

CBT can be a very helpful tool in treating mental health disorders, such as depression, PTSD, or an eating disorder. But not everyone who benefits from CBT has a mental health condition. It can be an effective tool to help anyone learn how to better manage stressful life situations.

I have heard great things about EMDR, a psychotherapy treatment that was originally designed to alleviate the distress associated with traumatic memory. According to the EMDR Humanitarian Assistance Programs website, EMDR therapy is an eight-phase treatment which comprehensively identifies and addresses experiences that have overwhelmed the brain's natural resilience or coping capacity, and have thereby generated traumatic symptoms and/or harmful coping strategies. Through EMDR therapy, patients are able to reprocess traumatic information until it is no longer psychologically disruptive.

Psychopharmacology is also an effective way to treat anxiety, depression and/or trauma. However, it is well-documented that psychopharmacology alone is not as beneficial as combining it with psychotherapy. In other words, popping a pill and expecting a miracle isn't the best way to deal with things. Popping a pill *and* regularly seeing a therapist is more evidence-based and will produce better outcomes. That didn't come out right but I think you get the gist.

There are many different types of antidepressants, antipsychotics, anti-anxiety and mood stabilizing medications. In my opinion and experience, do not rely on your family physician to prescribe these medications. Go to a psychiatric nurse practitioner or psychiatrist. They are well-versed in what works best for each person's situation and body chemistry.

Ask about genetic testing to see which medications to try and which to avoid for your genetic body type. Since these medications are heavily metabolized by the liver's cytochrome P450 pathway, genetic mutations of this pathway's liver enzymes can predict which psychiatric medications will work best for you. I have never tolerated a certain type of antidepressant and after getting that genetic consult I talked about previously it made sense. My genetic mutations equated to me being a rapid metabolizer of this type of drug.

If you want to steer clear of pharmaceuticals, you could stick with therapy or seek a consult with a natural health practitioner. He or she may be able to treat your condition with supplements, herbs, or diet. There are many ways to tackle anxiety and depression with natural treatments.

Physical Exercise

For some SOD patients, physical exercise triggers SOD symptoms. I have had this personally happen to me numerous times when I engaged in high interval training exercises. A few other people in the support groups complained of the same thing. Every time they ran or did aerobics they would have an SOD attack. It is sad to read how some SOD patients have had to give up competitive racing and sports or limit physical activities they loved because of the resulting SOD flares.

Please do not perform an exercise that will bring on pain. It isn't worth it. I know it is hard to give up something you love but it is also horrible and traumatic to deal with severe pain. That puts a lot of unhealthy stress on the body and mind. It is well known that pain increases blood pressure and can even cause shock. Quite a few SOD patients have reported passing out from SOD pain. Instead, find a healthy activity with the benefits of cardiovascular and muscle toning but doesn't leave you screaming in pain. Work on finding treatments that help your SOD symptoms and then reintroduce high impact exercises gradually.

There are many varieties of activities you could try. I started hiking again. My parents were avid hikers so I grew up hiking mountains and trails. I bought a quality pair of hiking boots so I wouldn't be in pain from sore feet. Quality footwear for any exercise or physical activity is important and worth the investment. People with SOD seem to do well with yoga. There are all sorts of yoga. You can pick and choose from gentle to more advanced or even hot yoga where you perform yoga in a heated room.

Bicycling may be a good activity for SOD sufferers. I just wouldn't recommend an intense spinning class if you want to avoid flare-ups. Brisk walking and swimming are other great ways to get a full body workout without putting too much stress on your body. Whatever you do, get off that couch and try something! Of course, if you were as sick as me during my worst year, I was too weak to do much of anything and couldn't afford to lose weight from exercising. If this is the case, stick with very gentle stretching or Tai Chi.

Spiritual Support

Whether you are an atheist, agnostic or deeply religious person, strengthening your spiritual condition will most certainly benefit you. For atheists or agnostics, you may feel spiritual by taking the time to be with nature or quieting the mind through meditation. If you are religious or feel a devotion to a particular religion or school of thought, think about increasing your attendance and presence at your religion's or spiritual practice's gathering place. Get involved in prayer groups or let people know you need prayers. I firmly believe the power of prayer contributed to me getting well again. I had so many people praying for me—friends, family, church members, and even strangers on Facebook. I don't know how to describe it other than I "felt" the love and now that I am better believe prayers helped me.

If you are too sick or exhausted to leave the house, you can watch religious services online. You'd be surprised how many different types of religious services you can attend right from the comfort of your own couch or bed. Some worldwide churches have cell phone apps to watch services and deliver special messages. I have satellite radio in my car and often listen to some of the religious/spiritual channels.

Pick up a devotional book or daily meditation that is religious or spiritual. You can also find these geared specifically for people with chronic pain and illness. The most important thing is that you find something that will reinforce positive messages and an attitude of faith and hope. I find starting my day off reading a daily meditation from my spiritual practice started the day off much better than when I forgot to read it.

Something else to consider is Chronic Pain Anonymous. It is a wonderful 12-step spiritual, not religious program, for people with chronic pain *and* chronic illness. There aren't many face to face in-person meetings but they have at least one phone or online meeting every day. Their website is www.chronicpainanonymous.com. Through the therapeutic value of support and the 12 steps (adopted from programs like Alcoholics Anonymous and Narcotics Anonymous), you can learn to cope and live with chronic pain and chronic illness. The cornerstone of 12-step programs like this is "working" spiritual principles like surrender, acceptance, honesty, willingness, etc.

Stop Going to Doctors

At some point, doctors may be doing more harm than good. If all you seem to be doing is going to doctors and hospitals, obsessing over a diagnosis and/or cure and going bankrupt as a result, consider taking a short break from it all. Obviously, if you need to head to the emergency room, do it. But, if you are exhausted like I was from constantly seeing doctors, most of whom were unable to help or refused to help me, treated me as an annoyance, and refused to go the extra mile to figure out how to best help me, then it may be wise to consider a little break.

I actually had some great moments of wellness when I stuck to natural remedies and practitioners, stayed off the Internet and rescheduled all my specialist appointments for a month or two later. Instead, I spent that extra time resting, attending group meditations at the local Buddhist center, got pedicures and manicures, started crocheting, and binge-watched some television shows. It was as if I took a vacation from being sick and, most importantly, from worrying about being sick and getting pissed off at doctors. Obviously, at some point I needed to see the doctor again, but the respite from all things medical was lovely.

Dealing with Financial Implications

The majority of SOD patients continue to work and excel in their career field. For 13 years, I climbed the ranks of a statewide advocacy organization, earning several promotions and recognition as a nationally known expert in children's mental health and juvenile justice family engagement and involvement. The entire time I had SOD. I would go to conferences and out to dinner with funders and policymakers, only to retreat to my hotel room in pain. I learned to live with it and not let it get in the way of any part of my life, including my career.

God was definitely on my side when I changed jobs in 2010. My new employer offered a long-term disability plan which I could have cared less about at the time of my hire. I was healthy and never thought I would ever need it. Boy was I wrong. In May 2012, after nine months of barely keeping it together at work because of the severity of my SOD symptoms, I decided to take a leave of absence. By August 2012, I was able to comfortably leave my position thanks to that long term disability policy. It enabled me to collect 60% of my income. The insurance company then forced me to apply for social security disability so they could collect their share. I received it on my first try.

I strongly encourage anyone with mild symptoms to get a long term disability policy as soon as possible. Do not hesitate. See if you can get one—no matter what the cost—that will pay out for pre-existing conditions. Contact your human resources department to see if they offer such a policy through your employer or search online for insurance companies that offer it. It is well worth the cost.

If you are already unable to work, consult with a social security disability attorney. Let them do the work of getting you qualified. The key to social security or any disability program is to have the support of your doctors. I would make office appointments with my physicians specifically to complete the forms required to document that I was disabled and unable to work. Do not think your doctors will fill these forms out just because they received them. Not one of my doctors voluntarily completed these forms. I had to persist. My primary care doctor and his staff have been amazing with getting documents submitted. However, the specialists required extra nudging.

When it is time to enroll in a health care plan at work, be sure to pick the best plan for inpatient and emergency room copays. One year, we had insurance where every inpatient copay was $1,000. I was in the hospital at least ten times so do the math. It was awful. Another year, we had a plan where I had to pay a copay for everything—every blood draw, scan, imaging study, procedure, etc. If I had all the money spent on health care since 2011 I'd have a brand new Lexus in the driveway and would have taken a trip around the world. At least I am alive and healthy. Things could certainly be worse.

Some say work and their careers kept them going through the worst SOD experiences. Others claim work made their symptoms worse. Whatever the case, explore all financial options that can support you when you need to heal and recover. Be prepared for the worst even if it never happens. Some in the U.S. utilize the Family Medical Leave Act (FMLA) to take short leaves of absence from their jobs. FMLA does not ensure you will get paid during that time but is supposed to protect you from losing your job. Caregivers can apply for FMLA as well if they need to care for you.

Be Kind to Yourself

I had to learn to be kind to myself throughout my illness. I had to stop saying things to myself I would never think of saying to another person. I'd get in a sickness rut and tell myself I was a loser, terrible wife and mother, hopeless, etc. I had to put post-it notes around my house telling me I would be ok, that I was a good person and other positive affirmations. I read a great book called, "The Anatomy of Hope," about people who never gave up hope no matter how grim their circumstance. I recommend it.

I had to quit the scale. I'd obsess over my drastic weight loss, weighing myself several times a day, driving myself crazy if I lost a pound. The fear of wasting away was awful. The actual wasting away was awful too. I was so thin I despised the way I looked. In time I learned to stop weighing myself, found clothes that flattered my shrinking body, and began to have acceptance about my situation and not look at the scale. I admit a small part of me still fears losing weight again, so I keep a supply of four different sizes of clothing in my closet. I am not ready to let this go just yet, which is ok.

It was costly buying a wardrobe every four to six months as I lost and re-gained weight. The best thing I learned was to rely heavily on thrift stores and friend's hand me downs. You would not believe the deals I found and the designer clothes people donate to places like the Salvation Army and Goodwill. I once found a hundred-dollar pair of designer Miss Me jeans for $3.99! For erratic weight loss and weight gain, hit the local thrift store. Or, let your friends know you are in need of clothing donations. Since most of my friends were bigger than my tiny frame, I accepted donations from their teenage and college-age daughters and ended up looking quite hip in American Eagle, Hollister, and Abercrombie and Fitch.

Getting off the Internet will help you to recover. I was obsessed with trying to figure out what was wrong with me to the point I couldn't stop searching the Internet. Although doing Internet research helped me get better and enabled me to write this book, I often went incredibly overboard with the amount of time I spent online, something my mom routinely commented on. Limit the time you spend online and stick to it! Spending an entire day on the Internet is not necessary and will only frustrate and scare you.

The television became both my best friend and my enemy, depending on the day and mood. I was couch- and bed-bound for so long that I ran out of things to watch. I can't believe some of the trash I watched. The worst were reality or talk shows where everyone looked perfect and had really stupid problems (in comparison to my life-threatening problems). I feared I'd never be right again and watching very rich people looking healthy, beautiful, and distraught over petty things pissed me off and made me feel worse. These shows were like train wrecks I couldn't help but watch. The best thing I figured out was to force myself to watch comedies—any comedy television show or movie—until I found one that made me laugh. Laughter truly can be the best medicine. I admit I still watch reality television but at least I don't feel pathetic anymore about my life.

Take up a hobby. I started crocheting again and am so glad I did. Making crocheted items has become a great way to give back to people who have helped me. I even make things for my doctors and their nursing staff. A popular hobby many are taking up is adult coloring books. They have great designs and patterns to choose from. You can use crayons, markers, or colored pencils. Walk into any craft store and you'll find an endless array of hobby items and kits to purchase, ex.jewelry making kits, calligraphy, needlepoint, scrapbooking, painting, drawing, weaving, etc.

Stick with Positive People

I am fortunate and grateful I have a husband who never doubted I would get better. He had enough faith and hope for about ten sick people. My mother, father, and stepparents did whatever they could to support and comfort me. Friends came and went. I had to routinely examine friendships. For the most part, I had supportive friends who stuck by my side. Some couldn't seem to deal with my illness or just went on with their busy lives. I am glad they showed this trait as I realized the hard way how valuable good, faithful friends were. I don't need unsupportive people in my life and neither do you.

I am blessed. Unfortunately, not everyone can say the same. I have watched many SOD patients lose spouses, friendships, and family members because these people couldn't handle the illness. The best thing you can do is put yourself and your health recovery first. Recognize that some losses end up being a Godsend. One woman who went through a horrible time with SOD, ERCPs, and surgery, had a husband cheat on her and walk out on her only a few months after she had major surgery. It was painful to read, but the good news was that his leaving was a positive thing. She recovered from SOD, healed emotionally, and is now in a much better relationship.

Set boundaries with toxic people. Obviously, for some of you this will be difficult as the toxic person could be your spouse, child, or other close family member. Therefore, I am not saying you go and divorce your husband or wife or disown family members. Learn to set healthy boundaries with a therapist or attend Al-anon if the toxic person is an addict or alcoholic.

Find positive and supportive people at church, in a support group, or through a hobby. I joined a small knitting group and the women became a huge source of support. I didn't even knit! I crocheted but they accepted me and I made great friendships.

For Caregivers, Family, and Friends

It takes a very self-centered individual to abandon someone who is ill and in need of support. For those of you reading this book as a caregiver, friend, or family member of an SOD patient, thank you for hanging in there. I know it isn't easy and at times overwhelming. My heart goes out to you.

You may wonder how you can be most helpful to someone with SOD. Being a nonjudgmental supporter is the best thing you can offer someone with SOD. Validate his or her symptoms and ask how you can help them through this difficult time. If they have a hard time asking for help, offer to run an errand, watch a child, accompany him or her to a doctor's appointment or procedure (this is by far one of *the* most helpful things you can do), or cook a meal they can actually eat. Anything that takes stress off him or her is helpful. Some SOD sufferers need someone to be their voice at doctor's appointments and emergency room visits as not all medical professionals understand or know about SOD. Having an advocate on board boosts a patient's chances of getting adequate treatment.

If you play a significant role as a caregiver, be sure to take care of yourself. It can be frustrating and oftentimes depressing to be the caregiver of a person with SOD. My husband and entire family were saints throughout my health nightmare. The best thing I could do as the sick person was push them to do fun things even if I had to stay home. They had every right to enjoy life. Caregivers shouldn't be expected to stay home every time we do. Sometimes pushing myself to do things with my husband, kids, friends, or family was the best gift I could give them. I didn't have to be on top of my game. I just needed to be there.

Caregivers can also try creative ways to bring happiness and fun to the SOD patient stuck in bed or on the couch. Watch a movie together. Read a book or magazine to them. Listen to an audio book together. Play a board or card game. Color or paint together. Do a jigsaw puzzle. The possibilities are endless.

Chapter 11: Emergency Rooms and Hospitals

Most of you will experience SOD symptoms yet never enter a hospital except to get bloodwork, a scan, or an outpatient procedure. The rest of you will have occasional or frequent trips to the emergency room (ER) coupled with inpatient hospital stays. For an entire year spanning 2011 to 2012, hospitals were my second home. ERs were my frequent stomping grounds. Therefore, I thought it fitting to include an entire chapter about them.

Trust me, I would have much rather been at a concert, swimming in a lake, or hanging out with my family and friends than spending my days and evenings in a hospital. I look back now and wonder how I made it through that time in my life. It was beyond depressing and miserable. Hospitals are necessary for certain issues but they sure aren't four-star hotels or a day spa. Some are better than others, though. You may want to make the rounds around town to see which hospital and ER you feel most comfortable in, especially if you are beginning to be a frequent flier at the ER.

There were a few times I drove an extra 40 minutes north to the hospital my mom worked at because it had the cleanest, newest, and nicest atmosphere; and, frankly, had the most attentive and caring staff. I would take the extra drive even though I had three other hospitals to choose from within a ten-minute drive.

In the beginning, I thought all hospitals and ERs were the same. Whichever one was closest would do. The first time I went to an ER for my SOD, it was an uneventful experience. I had been severely nauseous for several days and could not stop dry heaving and vomiting. At the local ER, I was treated well and had bloodwork and other tests. My subsequent visits weren't always so easy and pleasant. I boycotted that hospital when the GI doctors and staff there started to treat me as though my symptoms were entirely psychological. I haven't been there since 2011. I am blessed to have the choice of seven hospitals within a 35-mile radius but some aren't worth going to unless I have a severed limb. Even then I'm not sure how I'd be treated.

Over the course of a year, I spent roughly 100 days in and out of the hospital. As such, I became an "expert" hospital patient. Here are some suggestions if you need to go to the ER or hospital.

Have Your Doctor Call Ahead

Prior to going to the ER, visit your primary care doctor or gastro-enterologist or call to tell them you are having severe symptoms. Ask them to call the ER in advance of your arrival. The doctor should tell the ER staff he or she is recommending you be seen and treated. Possibly they could help you to get admitted as an inpatient if symptoms are severe. Your doctor may also recommend specific tests and give a brief history to the ER staff of why you need to be seen. In some hospitals, doing this may fast track you past some of the other less serious ER patients. It will also help ensure you are taken seriously if your tests come back normal.

Bring Information about SOD

Most emergency room staff are not knowledgeable about SOD or they know very little about our condition unless you go to a hospital where SOD doctors practice. Some SOD patients have told me bringing a one-page information sheet on SOD has helped doctors and nurses understand their condition. Most medical professionals will appreciate this information. Alternatively, I've heard of people with other diseases ordering fold over business cards with information about their disease on them. This is a great idea. There are several websites, like Vistaprint (http://www.vistaprint.com/), where you can design your own bookmarks, business cards, postcards, etc. at an affordable price. You can get ideas of what information to provide from the SODAE Network website (http://www.sodae.org).

Go to the Hospital Where your Gastroenterologist is Affiliated

Most gastroenterologists are affiliated with a specific hospital. Some have offices and clinics in the hospital. All should have a hospital of preference where they perform all of their outpatient procedures like a colonoscopy and endoscopy. When you arrive at the ER, be sure to inform the staff you are a patient of Dr. _____. Ask your doctor in advance, during an office visit or in writing, to make sure he or she writes out directives ahead of time for hospital staff to access your electronic medical records. These directives should provide general recommendations on how ER staff should treat you if you are to end up there. For example, your doctor can recommend specific pain control and a hydration protocol.

Be Prepared for an Inpatient Stay

Remember those old "Going to Grandma's" bags? When I was going through that period of time when my illness landed me in the hospital frequently and unexpectedly, I had a special hospital bag packed and ready to go at all times. Bring this bag with you anytime you go to the ER (you could get admitted as an inpatient), have an outpatient procedure (because you never know if you'll end up staying overnight), or when you know you will be in the hospital overnight. Pack the following items:

Clothes: Sweatpants, camisole or jogging bra (for women), tank top undershirt (for men or women), and multiple pairs of underwear. You could bring shorts or sweatpants but the hospital likely won't let you wear them as they will need to occasionally perform abdominal exams and the elastic band will get in the way.

If you are underweight like I was, you will want something to wear underneath the gown as the gowns the hospitals provide are designed for an incredibly large person. I begged for child-size gowns but it always fell on deaf ears. It certainly wouldn't hurt to have your nurse call the pediatric ward for a gown preferably meant for a medium- or large-sized child.

Non-slip socks or slipper socks: These are usually provided by the hospital, but they are thin and not as comfy as the fluffy kind you can buy yourself.

Toothbrush and toothpaste: Not essential as hospitals generally provide these, but if you have a favorite toothbrush and toothpaste, there isn't any harm in having them on hand.

Trial size hair and body products: I doubt you will want the cheap brands of hair care and body products the hospital will give you. You can buy those empty travel containers advertised in the drug store meant for air travel carry-ons. Fill each of them with your favorite shampoo, conditioner, and body wash. I would be so ill upon entering the hospital that I wouldn't be able to shower for several days. I'd feel so icky by the time I took a shower, but the smell of my body and hair care products gave me instant comfort, like a mini spa. They also reminded me of home.

Eye mask and ear plugs: These are not to be overlooked essentials. You will thank me if ever you are stuck having to share a hospital room with a loud snorer or the shades don't work and sunshine is streaming in, blinding you. You will be in a hospital for the purpose of rest and recovery. These two items will help you achieve that. If you forget these or get to the hospital and realize you want these, the neurology department of any hospital typically has them on hand. Ask your nurse to work on getting you them. If they tell you they don't have them, ask them to check with the neurology wing.

Things to keep you occupied: Pack reading material (magazines, books, an electronic tablet), puzzle books, headphones, or anything else to keep busy. These items are for when you start to feel better and are awaiting discharge. Keep in mind that if you can read and go on your tablet or phone, chances are you will be looked at as NOT an emergency or seriously ill. These items are also great if you are stuck waiting to have a procedure or surgery.

Medications: Technically, once you are admitted to a hospital or ER you are not supposed to take your own medications. However,

I went many days and nights without important medications due to doctor oversight or the hospital ran out. Yes, the hospital ran out of my medications! The problem was if I skipped even a day without a certain medication, I'd have severe vertigo to the point I'd fall over.

Another medication came with a seizure risk if I missed a dose. No one seemed to take this seriously. So many things can go wrong at the hospital from when the doctors order medications to when the nurses hand them out to you during medication rounds. I have witnessed too many instances where patients have actually had seizures because they didn't get their meds in a timely manner—instances where this could have been prevented. I don't think we should violate hospital rules but I also don't think we should end up with a seizure or other awful side effect when it could have been avoided.

My experience is that ERs want you treated and out of there or admitted into the hospital. They don't want to be worried about dispensing your usual meds unless it is life threatening. Long and short of it is I got in the habit of bringing my meds to any ER visit, procedure, or hospital stay. I would let the hospital staff know I had them just in case I needed them. On a few occasions, they gave me permission to self-medicate.

On other occasions, the hospital held onto my meds and doled them out to me from my supply. I don't know if this was legal or within hospital policy, but it got me through. Whatever you do, do NOT ever bring medications with you and not be honest about taking them while in the ER or hospital. You could take something, fall asleep, and get an IV dose by a nurse, causing a bad reaction or even an overdose. Always discuss medications with the hospital staff.

The Dreaded NPO

For many SOD patients, medications may not be an issue if you are "NPO." In that case, you have no choice but to rely on the hospital to administer your medications intravenously. NPO translates to "Nil per os", which is Latin for "nothing by mouth". It is a medical instruction to withhold oral intake of food and fluids. Doctors will order this for several reasons. The most common reason is to try to give your digestive system a rest. Those with acute pancreatitis often have to go NPO for several days and sometimes weeks.

Resting the pancreas is supposed to help it recover from an inflammatory attack. NPO will also be ordered if you cannot stop vomiting. The doctor will want to get the vomiting and nausea under control before food is reintroduced. Sometimes NPO was easy, especially if I had horrendous nausea. Other times it was torture, hence why I referred to it as "dreaded." Though I was sick, to not eat for several days left me starving. One time I had a hospital roommate whose family brought her Kentucky Fried Chicken. I was starving (hadn't eaten in three days), and it smelled so good. It was awful. It infuriated me that she was allowed to eat it in front of me like that.

Be careful when coming off NPO. You may feel like eating a very large meal and even feel well enough to eat a four-course meal. Whatever you do, do not believe the lies your cravings are telling you. Yes, you are hungry, but you are still sick and eating too much will set you back. Start with broth, Jell-O, toast, and slowly advance with extremely small portions. Whatever you do, don't sneak food or beverages behind your doctor's back. Only ingest what they say you can ingest.

No or Very Few Visitors

I could not for the life of me understand why people in the hospital need a large group of people visiting them. I can understand if you just had a baby, but if you are in the hospital for SOD that means your symptoms are severe and you need rest, not a party. I got in the habit of telling my friends I only wanted family visiting, which they understood. If you are up to having a small get-together in your hospital room, playing cards, and having a grand old time catching up, then you probably don't even need to be in the hospital and are wasting money, people's time, and a valuable hospital bed someone else may need. It is perfectly ok to tell people not to visit you. You need the rest and need to get well, not have a mini cocktail party or family reunion.

I am not talking about your parents, kids and spouse popping by. I am talking about the hospital roommates who would have visitor after visitor from morning till late at night. No one seemed to abide by the visiting hours at any hospital I'd ever been a patient. None of the nursing staff enforced it, that was for sure. I had hospital roommates with visitors disturbing me at midnight! I did get in the habit of asking to be switched to another room. I'd complain enough to where it would happen.

Take Advantage of Alternative Therapies

Hospitals nowadays offer many different complementary therapies to help make your stay a comfortable one. I have taken advantage of reiki, pet therapy, and massages during hospital stays. Other therapies a hospital may offer are music and art therapy, guided imagery or meditation, relaxation training, and acupuncture. For me, the best was the pet therapy. It really was therapeutic being able to pet a nice friendly dog while in a hospital bed. Ask your nurse if the hospital offers any of these things.

Fight the "Drug Seeker" Label

A common problem I and many other SOD and pancreatitis sufferers experienced was being treated as a drug seeker. Since many of us have normal bloodwork and scans, emergency room doctors and staff are more likely to treat us as though we are faking our pain to get narcotic pain medication. We don't have a body part that is broken show up on a scan or blood oozing from every orifice. Unless our pancreatic enzyme levels are extremely high, it may be difficult convincing ER staff of the pain you are in. We know our pain is real and during a severe attack the last thing we want to have to worry about is convincing the medical profession it is indeed real. Unfortunately, more times than not I'd be treated like a drug seeker in the ER as I was moaning in pain for hours without relief.

At first, I didn't fight being treated this way. I didn't have it in me. I knew I wasn't in the ER or hospital to get drugs and that was all that mattered. However, one time I was in horrific pain and an ER doctor proceeded to lecture me on the dangers of opioid medication rather than treat my pain. The friend who accompanied me to the ER and I didn't know what to make of it. I hadn't even asked for any drugs; I was simply a patient in pain. At that point, I took a stand and told him to just treat me (with a few swear words thrown in).

Don't put up with this. If a nurse or doctor makes a snarky remark about pain meds or insinuates you are seeking drugs and may have an addiction issue, ask for the hospitalist. The hospitalist is there to ensure you get adequate care and are treated with dignity. If the hospitalist does not help you, ask for someone who can and let them know you will be reporting them to the Joint Commission. It is a fact that when attacks are very bad, SOD patients may require pain medication. Unfortunately, in this day and age, it is difficult convincing doctors as such.

Read Your Discharge Papers Thoroughly

Ask for your medical records/papers associated with your discharge prior to leaving the hospital. Thoroughly review what the attending physician wants you to do once you leave the hospital. He or she may have already set up an appointment with one of your regular doctors as a follow-up or may have suggested you see a new doctor for a consult. They may have prescriptions for you to have filled or may have sent them electronically to your pharmacy. Be sure to ask any questions you have about medications, including dosage and side effects.

Do not sign anything that states anything negative about you from your visit to the ER or hospital stay. Anything said goes in your permanent file. If a doctor writes that you are a difficult patient, the next doctor who treats you at your next ER visit will see this. I can't tell you how many women have written in our support groups that they received copies of their records only to find a doctor wrote they came to the ER seeking drugs, which was likely a false accusation. I doubt all of these women with painful SOD are solely going to the ER for drugs.

Some of you reading this may think I am exaggerating or sensationalizing this topic but trust me that it is happening everywhere and more and more frequently. You must formally request this information be removed from your records. You do not want this on your permanent record. Every future doctor will see this. It could even prevent you from trying to get life or disability insurance policies.

As a final note, please only go to the hospital if you absolutely cannot manage things at home. There were a few times I could have stayed home but I actually wanted to go to the hospital to be forced with NPO and get some IV hydration. As a result, I ended up getting unnecessary scans and was exposed to a highly contagious bacterium called c difficile (c diff), which produced the worst diarrhea you can imagine and took a month to eradicate. Too often, I hear of SOD patients contracting the flu, virus, c diff, or some other illness from going to the hospital. Stay home, but if you do have to go to the hospital keep your hands and possessions clean.

Chapter 12: Be an Empowered Patient

In the beginning of my health journey, I prided myself on trying to be a model patient. Whatever I was facing, health-wise, I had faith my doctors would help me. I believed that they believed in me and wanted to help me. I don't doubt every doctor wants the best for their patients. But, over time I learned through pain and misery that not every doctor I saw was capable of helping me. Some developed opinions of me which impeded their ability to treat me. Others simply did not have the tools or knowledge to help me with this condition. And, others were closed-minded to the concept of SOD. Fortunately, throughout my health journey, I experienced a paradigm shift. I went from being a model, meek patient to an empowered, vocal patient.

I can bitch and moan about the terrible doctor experiences I've had but one thing I learned about myself was that my expectations of doctors were often unrealistic. If every doctor, nurse, or other healthcare provider is a problem to you, then it's probably your expectations that need to be adjusted and not necessarily the healthcare provider's behaviors that are the problem. That isn't to say you are in the wrong 100%. I simply doubt every single provider is to blame. Even though a large majority of doctors I saw were a disappointment, there were a few I cannot say didn't have my best interest in mind and it showed in their care, concern, compassion, and willingness to go the extra mile for me. I acknowledged them at the beginning of this book.

At some point along my journey, I developed a zero-faith attitude toward the healthcare system and its providers. Looking back, I realize many were acting the way they were out of frustration. Here I was clearly very ill and yet they, the health professional, could not figure out how to help me. I had one doctor tell me, "I got into medicine to help people and successfully treat patients. It doesn't seem like you will ever get better, which goes against why I became a doctor." For quite some time, I was infuriated by his comment. In fact, I never saw this doctor again. Today, I understand what he was trying to tell me. The delivery sucked, but I believe he wished me well.

Possibly, expectations about doctors were engrained in my mind throughout my life. I think most people grow up thinking doctors are God-like. I was no different. I always figured, the rule of life was that I'd go to the doctor if my children or I was sick and my doctor would "fix" us. Usually fixing meant writing a prescription. So, when I became so ill I could barely function, I developed an intense anger toward the medical profession when they failed me. How could they not help me? Why were they not believing me? Why were they not doing the legwork to refer me to a doctor who *could* help me? It was a hopeless and lonely feeling.

As time went on and I didn't get better, I developed resentments with just about every doctor I saw. Even my beloved primary care doctor got blamed for my pain and nausea. I was especially irritated when he refused to treat my pain though I was ready to jump off a bridge from the pain being so bad. Aside from my father, brother, and oldest son, he was the longest relationship I had with a man (20+ years). Fortunately, I got over it and carry no ill will against him today. He is still my primary care doctor.

I made many mistakes along the way and could write an entire book on how to become an empowered patient. Luckily, there are dozens of these books already written. If you want to read an entire book on becoming an empowered patient, I recommend two books: "The Take-Charge Patient: How You Can Get the Best Medical Care" by Martine Ehrenclou and "The Empowered Patient: How to Get the Right Diagnosis, Buy the Cheapest Drugs, Beat Your Insurance Company, and Get the Best Medical Care Every Time" by Elizabeth S. Cohen. I have read these books and believe every patient should read them.

It Is Ok to Move On or Fire a Doctor

As I said, I made many mistakes. I cannot blame all of my woes on doctors or the healthcare system. The first mistake I made was relying too heavily on my local doctors and their schedules. By the time I made it out to the SOD specialist in Minnesota, where I finally got diagnosed and treated the first time, I had already wasted away to 95 pounds and was profoundly weak and disabled. I spent nearly a year putting all my faith into the local doctors. I was certain they would fix me and having to wait long periods in between appointments and tests was standard. Looking back, there were clear signs from the beginning they couldn't or wouldn't fix me, but I felt like I would be a bad patient for jumping ship. How wrong I was!

These doctors thought it was perfectly ok for me to continue waiting months between appointments and tests, though my symptoms and health took a nosedive quickly. I will never wait on doctors again. Please, especially if you are losing weight at a dangerous rate, do NOT waste your time with any doctor who does not treat this as an urgent life-threatening manner. I honestly think they believed I was anorexic, mentally ill, or that whatever I had would go away soon. If I had to do over again, after the first few months of getting nowhere locally, I would have traveled to that SOD specialist in Minnesota much sooner. If he wasn't able to help me I would have found another doctor and so on.

Most of the doctors I no longer see don't even know I fired them. I just never went back to them. There is no need to inform them of your plans to move on. Simply sign a release so your new doctors can access your medical records. I don't go around firing every doctor who doesn't meet every need. That would be reckless. I do get rid of doctors who have bad bedside manners, aren't compassionate, won't perform testing, are close-minded to alternative treatments, make me wait more than an hour repeatedly, and aren't thorough.

Bring an Advocate

The second mistake I made was not bringing along a good advocate to my appointments. My mom, who is an operating room nurse, would accompany me to nearly every appointment. She provided an incredible source of comfort and support. That poor woman went through as much hell as I did. However, my mom is very much of the old-school belief that the doctor knew best—at least in most cases. With the urgency of my condition, I really needed someone to put their foot down with doctors, especially the GI doctor who could have performed an ERCP right here in my hometown.

Regretfully, I should have engaged my husband in all of my healthcare appointments. It wasn't that he didn't want to attend my appointments. We couldn't afford to have him miss work, especially since I was about to lose my ability to work due to my health. I noticed that the rare occasions my husband attended doctor appointments with me, doctors listened to him. This was especially true with doctors of certain cultures. It is a reality that in some cultures, women are to be talked to, not heard from. I witnessed this.

One local GI doctor who dropped the ball with me did not do the same for male patients I knew. Worse than not bringing a vocal advocate was when I would go alone to appointments. That was a huge mistake. I was definitely dismissed more readily when I was alone. Bring someone, anyone, you know with good advocacy skills. Bring your spouse, parent, adult child, friend, church member, or basically anyone, but don't go alone.

Be Strong

I was so sick and frightened over my illness that I'd cry at every office visit. This reaffirmed to the doctors I had mental health issues and not a real disorder. I know it is depressing to be sick and difficult to not cry every time you are in a doctor's office, but try your hardest to pull yourself together. It is ok to appear sick. You don't want to walk into a doctor's appointment or procedure all sunshine and rainbows or have perfect hair and makeup. If you do, I can guarantee your doctor won't see you as an urgent case. Be the sick person you are but try not to cry or at least not that ugly, sobbing cry. I could feel the exam room get tense when I'd start crying.

I think it makes doctors uncomfortable.

Read Those Office Notes and Records

Just as I advised to review your discharge papers from the ER or hospital, routinely ask for your medical records and office notes from your primary care doctor and all specialist appointments. I made the mistake of deciding a few years ago to read all of my medical records and office notes. Why was this a mistake? Because I should have been doing it all along and much sooner, not a year after my illness. Incredibly, there were many incorrect and defamatory statements written about me.

Unfortunately, I could not do anything about them as the records were a year or two old. I could not believe what I was reading. It was awful. The tone by the doctors or other healthcare workers in some of the office notes was nothing short of blaming and shaming the patient for being ill. If you come across anything you don't agree with, contact the doctor's practice and request the statement(s) be removed or changed.

Stand Up for Yourself

I had some wonderful nurses and doctors, but sadly I also had some awful nurses and doctors. Keep in mind, not everyone loves their jobs and that includes some nurses and doctors. Their attitudes and treatment can negatively affect your quality of care and impede your recovery. It is well-known that the nursing profession has a high burnout rate, and understandably so. The same holds true for some doctors. Burnout is a huge factor with long hours, but some may not even like their jobs.

In an online Medscape/WebMD questionnaire of 24,000 doctors representing 25 specialties, only 54%, said they would choose medicine again as a career. Just 41% would choose the same specialty again. Only a quarter of doctors said they would choose the same practice setting, compared with 50% a year prior. Why such frustration and discontent among physicians? The survey cites declining incomes, excessive paperwork, and vast uncertainty about changes dictated by the United States Affordable Care Act.

In my opinion, this survey was quite accurate. About half the medical staff I've encountered were great, compassionate, empathetic, caring, interested in my well-being, smart, and thorough. Resident doctors (doctors who completed medical school and were working on their final residency requirements) were almost always the best when it came to my care in hospitals. I guess they hadn't become jaded yet. I wish I could find them now to tell them how wonderful they treated me and to not lose sight of that quality.

Not every ER, hospital, or doctor's office experience will be entirely good or entirely bad. My hope for you is regardless of your experience, you will be an empowered patient. You will advocate for yourself and not tolerate substandard care. In the event you feel you need to make a formal complaint about a doctor or hospital, follow these suggestions (taken from Trisha Torrey's article, "Complain About a Doctor or Other Healthcare Provider").

Remember that everyone has an occasional bad day. But a pattern of mistakes, arrogance or misconduct which have resulted in detriment to a patient may mean that doctor or another provider should be reported to someone who can help affect change, or remove that provider from practice.

Always begin by complaining directly to the doctor who created the problem. If approaching the doctor directly doesn't get you anywhere, contact the practice manager and make a verbal report, followed by a letter or email that spells out your complaint and your expectations as discussed by phone.

As I mentioned in the "Finding an SOD Doctor" chapter, there are doctor rating sites. This is your opportunity to rate your doctor—negative or positive.

Be aware there will be ramifications if you make a formal complaint and the doctor knows you were the source. If you can find another doctor easily then that is not a big deal. But, if you are looking to preserve your relationship, be mindful a doctor can and will drop you. Patient abandonment is frowned upon but happens all the time.

Do not become that patient who complains about every doctor he or she meets. Doctors talk amongst themselves and any resistance will be duly noted in your medical records.

Even if the problem didn't take place in the hospital, find out what hospitals your doctor is affiliated with and complain to two of their personnel: 1. whoever is in charge of patient relations and 2. whomever is in charge of risk management. Call the hospital to ask for the names and mailing addresses of the people who hold those positions.

Complain to your local medical society. There is probably not much they can do, but if they begin to see a pattern about one doctor from many sources, they will contact the doctor and try to suggest some sort of correction. Find your local medical society by searching on the Internet for the phrase "medical society" and either your city, county or region name.

Complain to your doctor's medical board. You can tell which boards those are by looking up your doctor online, then finding the information about his training and certifications, such as "Board Certified by ____." Some boards have their own complaint procedures listed on their websites. If the board your doctor was certified by doesn't have a formal complaint procedure, then find an address on the "Contact us" page, and ask that it be delivered to someone who looks at disciplinary or revocation issues.

Complain to the Joint Commission. Hospitals fear The Joint Commission (https://www.jointcommission.org/) (formerly called JHACO) and do not want them knocking at their door. The Joint Commission is the organization that accredits hospitals and works toward improved safety for patients, among other hospital quality efforts. If your complaint is associated with an ER visit or hospital stay, you can submit a complaint online or in a letter.

Complain to your state's professional licensing bureau, medical board, and/or health or insurance department. Each state handles complaints about medical professionals differently.

Hopefully, you won't ever have to make a verbal or written complaint, but if you do, don't expect miracles to happen, apologies to be made, or acknowledgment of wrong-doing. Practice acceptance that you may never get justice for whatever happened or didn't happen. The point is your complaint could help the next person complaining or something may actually be done about the problem.

Chapter 13: If It Isn't SOD What Is Wrong with Me?

If you are unfortunate to have gone through SOD testing and treatments and still do not have a diagnosis, you may not have SOD. Though SOD is difficult to diagnose, all of the normal tests may be correct. It is even more difficult than ever to get an accurate SOD diagnosis as the once "gold standard" method for diagnosing SOD, ERCP with manometry, has been largely abandoned by many of today's gastroenterologists, mostly due to the outcomes of the EPISOD study (discussed in the next chapter) but also because it isn't entirely reliable, though it is the "gold standard." Therefore, you could very well have SOD though your doctor is telling you that you do not. Or, like I said earlier you may not have SOD and need to consider other possible causes for your symptoms.

What it Could Be

There is an actual condition called Medically Unexplained Physical Symptoms (MUPS). Fibromyalgia and Chronic Fatigue Syndrome used to be MUPS before they had names. You may have this or you may have something with an actual name. Regardless, the important thing is you take care of yourself and never give up searching for a diagnosis and relief from your symptoms. Here are a few possible causes to your "SOD-like" symptoms, i.e. upper right quadrant pain with or without nausea, vomiting, unintended weight loss, diarrhea, constipation, malnutrition, and/or pancreatic and liver abnormalities.

Biliary colic/spasm: The bile duct can spasm, causing pain. People I know with these issues get substantial relief from stents. Stents can control painful spasms and open the bile duct for bile to flow better. Antispasmodic medications, particularly long-acting, help some people too. The only way of knowing whether this is the cause of your symptoms is by experimenting with treatments to see if they work on the symptoms.

Biliary sludge: Bile is a liquid that shouldn't be thick and clumpy. Sludge is bile that contains microscopic gallstone crystals and is thick, which doesn't flow freely. This will give you unpleasant symptoms. I think anyone having an ERCP should ask their doctors to collect some bile and have it sent to a lab. There, the lab can look at it under a microscope to see if it indeed has gallstone crystals. They can also test to see if the bile is infected with bacteria.

I am quite fond of theories by a Russian doctor named Dr. Turumin (http://www.drturumin.com/en/PostCholecystectomySyn-drom_en.html). For biliary sludge and SOD, he promotes the use of Celecoxib (Celebrex) and Ursodeoxycholic acid (Ursodiol, Actigall) based on studies he conducted of post-cholecystectomy patients. Stents may be helpful too, but can get clogged rather quickly.

Papillary stenosis: This is narrowing around the sphincter. It can be triggered by trauma and inflammation due to pancreatitis, instrumentation (ex. ERCP), or prior passage of a stone. People who have had a successful sphincterotomy can experience stenosis with or without scar tissue months or years after the procedure. Treatment is balloon dilatation or repeat sphincterotomy via ERCP.

Motility Disorders: In an ideal scenario digestion occurs in a symbiotic regulated manner. Everything works like a big cog machine. However, anytime there is an assault on the digestive system, i.e. surgery, viruses, hormones, bacteria, fluid change, etc. this perfectly regulated system can be thrown off. Gastroparesis is an example of a motility disorder where stomach contents empty too slow. Depending on how sensitive a person is, even a slight change over time can result in disabling symptoms.

This is where a functional medicine practitioner would be helpful or an acupuncturist to "realign" your body. In regards to motility and nausea, as I mentioned in the medications chapter, domperidone helped me greatly. Other motility aids are bitters, an herbal concoction called Iberogast, or the prescription drug, metoclopramide. A gastroparesis diet can be helpful as well. Please know you can have a fairly normal gastric emptying study but still experience symptoms. There is an excellent book called, "Living Well with Gastroparesis (http://livingwithgastroparesis.com/)" by Crystal Zaborowski Saltrelli. I highly recommend it.

Bile reflux: Stagnant motility of the upper small intestine can result in bile refluxing into the stomach as can a problem with the stomach's pyloric valve, the valve that controls the emptying of stomach contents into the small intestine. Over time, bile acids can cause severe pain and nausea. Some doctors will prescribe a proton pump inhibitor or antacid, but there is no proof they work on bile, only stomach acid. A friend of mine with severe bile reflux gets relief with domperidone and Carafate. Some benefit from taking cholestyramine, a bile acid sequestrant, which also helps control bile diarrhea. Sleeping upright or at an angle can keep the bile down. A bed wedge is great for that. I got mine on Amazon and sleep on it every night.

Pancreas Issues: The pancreas can be an incredibly sensitive organ. Depending on the person, even a touch of chronic pancreatitis can cause moderate to severe pain, nausea, and loose stools. There are countless silent and invisible causes to chronic pancreatic inflammation, which is referred to as idiopathic chronic pancreatitis. Mystery causes can be from medications, biliary issues, autoimmune disorders, duct strictures, and hereditary or genetic predispositions. Prescription enzymes like Creon and Zenpep can help.

Medications: I can't tell you how many times I've had severe mystery ailments then stopped a medication and the symptoms completely abated. I even had doctors swear to me a medicine couldn't cause a symptom I had and yet it did. Check to see if a new or even old medication could be to blame. You could be the patient who has a rare 1% of the population side effect. We are all different. Cessation of a medication can also cause severe side effects. Many medications cause a withdrawal syndrome, not just addictive medications. Yes, medications *can* cause symptoms mimicking SOD.

Hormones: I don't think it is a coincidence the majority of SOD sufferers are women. I talk about hormones at length in the Causes of SOD chapter. To test and treat hormonal imbalance I had better luck seeing a functional medicine practitioner and naturopath than a gynecologist or my primary care doctor. The naturopath performed more detailed hormone testing than my regular doctor. I am currently being treated for low hormones and it has helped my digestion.

HPA axis dysfunction: The hypothalamic–pituitary–adrenal (HPA) axis is the system that makes sure our adrenals function correctly, which in turn affects our digestive system. It has been proven time and again that stress can contribute to digestive issues. Look on the Internet for "HPA axis and digestion." You will be surprised with what you read and how much this system affects you.

Conventional testing is generally useless unless your adrenals are in complete failure. A functional medicine practitioner or naturopath can do a saliva cortisol test to gauge cortisol readings throughout a given day. Things that help keep this system in balance are: avoiding sugar and processed foods, gentle exercise—not too much and not too little, avoiding stress, meditation, adrenal supplements, and adequate sleep.

Bacterial Dysbiosis: I see a lot of people's SOD symptoms flare after a round of antibiotics. After all, many antibiotics can cause pancreatitis! They can also cause a rebound overgrowth (small intestinal bacterial overgrowth, also known as SIBO). Bacteria control every aspect of digestion. If it is imbalanced your digestion will be as well. Treatments for this include more antibiotics, herbs, diet, and probiotics.

Food Intolerance: This is not to be confused with a food allergy. A food intolerance can cause many different symptoms or reactions and can be temporary or lifelong. Some food intolerances can produce SOD-like symptoms. As described in the SOD Diet chapter, keep a diligent food diary for several weeks by recording everything you drank and ate, supplements and medications you took, and activities like exercise. If you suffer from a food intolerance or other sensitivity, this should reveal itself as you keep track of foods, beverages, supplements, and medications. You may also find certain activities to be triggers.

Nerve/Rib Issue: If it is pain-only with no other symptoms, I would say investigate this as an option. If it is a nerve issue you will likely see an improvement in pain with nerve blocks or common nerve medications like gabapentin or Lyrica. A woman who was misdiagnosed with SOD shared that her pain all along was a slipped rib and is pain-free. I haven't seen research where a nerve or rib condition could cause nausea, vomiting, diarrhea, etc. unless the nerve and rib are somehow causing an obstruction. That is why if your only issue is the pain, definitely explore this as a possibility.

Cystic stump remnant syndrome: One theory that has been raised in our support groups and has been theorized by some doctors is the matter of the cystic duct remnant. Years ago, gallbladders were not removed laparoscopically. I remember when I was 14 years old, my best friend's sister had her gallbladder removed. She had a huge incision that kept her on the couch for over a month. She was in a tremendous amount of pain.

Back then, most, if not all, of the cystic duct was removed as it was easily done through open surgery. Since the risk of cutting the bile duct or another organ increases if the cystic duct is cut close during laparoscopic surgery, surgeons have opted to leave much of the duct hanging. One man posted in an SOD support group telling us he experienced complete relief of his SOD symptoms after a surgeon went in and shortened the remnant duct. This theory as a cause for SOD doesn't explain the high prevalence of female patients with SOD. But, it should be explored nonetheless. As stated earlier in this book, there is a bundle of nerves connecting the cystic duct with the bile duct and sphincters. If after CCK is released, the body attempts to contract a gallbladder that is no longer there, it may set off the cystic stump and all the nerves associate with it.

Liver disease and other conditions: There are many liver diseases that can cause SOD-like symptoms, ex. fatty liver disease, ascending and sclerosing cholangitis, and primary biliary cirrhosis. Though bloodwork or scans for these conditions are generally abnormal there are also cases where diseases are "silent" and difficult to detect.

SOD: Believe it or not, you can have normal bloodwork, scans, and even manometry and still have SOD. Your sphincters could be out of sync and not opening exactly when they are supposed to. You won't have a high-pressure spasm issue. Imagine instead that all of the sphincters are dysfunctioning, i.e. opening and closing improperly all at once? That would be one big hot mess! Sphincter spasm with elevated pressures isn't the only type of sphincter dysfunction.

What You Can Do

If you have been to specialist after specialist, consider taking a break from medical doctors, unless you think one of the previously mentioned medications or treatment options could help you or you would like further testing for liver or pancreas diseases.

If medical doctors have been thorough and you have been through extensive testing, find a good functional medicine practitioner and/or naturopath by searching online, asking friends and family, or ask your primary care doctor. You may have to interview a few before finding the right one. Ask if they are familiar with liver, biliary, and pancreatic issues.

Seek the consult of a good psychiatrist and mental health therapist for your mental health needs. As I've said before, if you didn't have mental health issues prior to getting sick, you now have them thanks to illness, fear of the unknown, and negative experiences with doctors.

Try acupuncture, hypnotherapy, reiki, yoga, meditating, or any other modality that could realign your digestive system and body energy field. Whatever you can do to de-stress those sphincters, ducts, and organs, do it. Get your body in balance again!

Re-evaluate the medications you are on and discuss tapering off any with your doctor. If your doctor recommends an antibiotic, ask about an alternative. More digestive issues begin because of antibiotics than anything else I've witnessed.

Be patient. I know this is easier said than done, but time is the best medicine for any condition. Think about it like this. You get a cold and continue to work, burn the candle at both ends, and wonder why after a month you can't get rid of the bronchitis that developed. If everyone stopped what they were doing when they got sick, practiced self-care and natural treatments, and relaxed, I guarantee most wouldn't be ill more than a week. Patience and time are important healers.

Don't give up and don't do this alone. I know how horrible and devastating it is to have unexplained symptoms. I truly do. Stick with people who believe in you and do not doubt your illness, that includes family and friends. Whatever it is that will get you out of the isolation of illness, do it!

Chapter 14: The Future of SOD

I was conflicted on how to end this book. Do I completely ignore the reality of what is happening with SOD as a diagnosis? Do I not mention the fact patients are being abandoned by their physicians, and researchers want to remove SOD as a diagnosis altogether? Should I turn a blind eye to doctors misdiagnosing SOD patients simply because they have a personal issue with or misinformed belief about SOD? Will keeping this book politically correct truly help the SOD patient?

The collective answer to all of these quandaries was, "Absolutely Not!" Glossing over the ugly truth about SOD and the horrible treatment of some patients would ultimately do more damage than good. After all, this is a survival guide, not "50 Positive Things About SOD." If we are to truly survive and have a quality of life with this difficult condition, we need to be validated and taken seriously by the doctors treating us.

A few days before putting the finishing touches on this book, I received a terrible email. A father wrote asking how people could donate to the SOD cause in lieu of flowers. His son had SOD and after a very bad flare up took his own life. This man's father wanted to know what is being done as far as research for SOD. This wasn't the first SOD-related tragedy I encountered and it certainly will not be the last, not unless SOD becomes a priority in the eyes of researchers, physicians, policymakers, and society as a whole.

I often wonder if there is a genetic component to this disease. If so, what if my granddaughter were to get this horrible disease? Would I be ok with her being treated the way I was treated? Absolutely not! We need comprehensive SOD research and awareness and we need it *now*.

SOD: A Public Health Reality

SOD is a health crisis that has gone unnoticed far too long. The

2014 SODAE Network patient survey summed up patient experiences as follows:

As a person with SOD, I currently struggle with (check all that apply)

Answer Options	Response Percent	Response Count
Chronic Pain	66.5%	127
Intermittent Pain	56.0%	107
Nausea and/or Vomiting	72.3%	138
Unintended Weight Loss	33.5%	64
Being Told My Condition is Psychological	34.6%	66
Health Care Workers' Lack of SOD Knowledge	71.7%	137
Finding a Doctor Who Treats SOD	51.3%	98
Finding a Treatment that Helps Symptoms	73.3%	140
Work, Family, Quality of Life Issues	75.4%	144
Lack of Compassion/Empathy from Family and	47.6%	91
Other (please specify)		24
answered question		191
skipped question		6

*Other specified were: Pancreatitis, Unintended Weight Gain, Diarrhea, Missing Work, Being Told "but you don't look sick", Trying to Explain SOD to People, Diet, Mounting Bills, Treated as a Drug Seeker, Being Misdiagnosed, Depression/Anxiety Over Being Sick, Fear of Next Attack, Diarrhea.

The socioeconomic effects of SOD can be summed up by analyzing the following information from the same survey:

In the past 12 months, how many times (for zero you will need to enter "1" this survey program won't allow zero or blanks)

Answer Options	Response Average	Response Total	Response Count
Did you visit an emergency room?	7.28	1,347	185
Were you an inpatient in the hospital	9.83	1,749	178
Did you miss work due to SOD (in days)? *	73.12	12,869	176
Did you visit a doctor--any doctor?	15.24	2,759	181
answered question			192
skipped question			5

The personal, financial, and societal impact of SOD is tragic. SOD patients miss out on life, lack financial security, and spend much of their lives in a mostly unsupportive medical system. The cost of SOD to insurance companies and governments is astronomical. Here is a rough cost analysis:

According to Kaiser State Health Facts, the average cost for one inpatient day in the hospital is $2,090. Applying the numbers above, it cost $3,148,200 in inpatient days for 192 SOD patients.

The Washington Post analyzed emergency room costs and determined the average cost per visit was $1,233, which translated to $1,660,851 for the 192 SOD patients' total ER visits. Add to the emergency room costs a CT scan, which is commonly performed every time an SOD patient enters an ER. The discrepancies in the cost of CT scans can range from $2,325 to $6,400 depending on which hospital you go to (source: New Choice Health). Take the average of that and a whopping $5,876,287 was potentially spent on these patients for CT scans. Do not forget to include the 2,759 office visits that can range from $200-$400 per visit--an approximate $827,700 total for our participants.

The total for all reported services listed above is $11,51,038. That equals $59,963 per patient each year. This is just the tip of the iceberg. We cannot even begin to actualize the cost for missed days of work, unemployment, and disability. Many SOD patients go into severe debt from the mounting copays. I calculated in one year from 2011-2012, my health insurance company paid out over $100,000 in claims. I paid about $15,000 in out of pocket copays.

By now we would expect an interest from the insurance companies and government to help advocate and coordinate care for SOD patients, and invest in SOD research. Though some insurance companies offer "care coordination", according to SOD patients, it is rarely helpful or effective. And, the research the U.S. government has invested in SOD is minuscule. These outcomes reinforce what we as patients know--that SOD is a public health crisis in dire need of attention at the local, national, and international levels. Moreover, the above results are not unique, mirroring the results of the previous year's survey.

Forget about the financial toll, which is obvious. The emotional toll and burden on not only the SOD patient but their families and friends, are immeasurable. We as patients do not need our diagnosis ripped away from us because a few researchers and doctors have formed opinions about us as patients and are, in my opinion, too closed-minded and unwilling to broaden their search for causes and treatments that make sense. We especially need to know why this is an overwhelmingly female-dominant disease.

Two months after I had my transduodenal sphincteroplasty, my surgeon told me at a follow-up appointment, "You know, they are discovering Sphincter of Oddi Dysfunction isn't real." After a pause of shock, I responded, "I'll have to disagree. How do you explain my sphincter pressures measured six times above the norm on the manometry scale? And, since the surgery, I no longer have 24/7 nausea and vomiting or severe right upper quadrant and that under-the-sternum pain."

In this doctor's defense, he was always very supportive and compassionate. He witnessed firsthand the suffering I endured from SOD. Deep down, he knew SOD was my affliction. I knew his statement did not come from a place of malice. He simply read or heard something and was repeating it to me. One of his good doctor buddies was the local GI doctor who refused to diagnose or treat me for SOD so he probably heard it from him.

Unfortunately, my doctor's comment about SOD was not an isolated incident. I read and listen to countless stories on a weekly basis of doctors telling patients that SOD (primarily SOD Type 3) does not exist. Many of our newest online support group members have asked their doctors to consider SOD as a diagnosis. The popular response from their GI doctors? "You don't have SOD," without any testing or trialing of SOD medications.

We are witnessing an epidemic in our community as too often those with SOD are abandoned by their doctors, and often told their symptoms are psychological or related to stress. What happens to these patients is they either exhaust their savings to travel far and wide to see a doctor who may or may not agree to help them or, those who cannot afford that option, are left with no treatment options and in time deteriorate physically and mentally.

I am not saying there couldn't be a psychological or stress component. There *was* a study published in 2016 of the antidepressant duloxetine (Cymbalta) showing an indication of efficacy in the treatment of pain in patients with suspected SOD, but adverse events limited its use and only about a dozen patients completed the study. Possibly, an antidepressant such as this assisted in mediating the patients' ability to cope with and tolerate the pain. It did not conclude whether it cured the primary issue or treated other disabling SOD symptoms like nausea.

A few years ago I happened to meet a gastroenterologist from Boston who repeated, almost verbatim, what my surgeon said—that SOD was not real! He heard this at a gastroenterology conference where the results of a U.S. National Institutes of Health study, Evaluating Predictors and Interventions in Sphincter of Oddi Dysfunction (EPISOD), were discussed. SOD has a history of being controversial, but this study pushed the controversy over the top, and not in a positive direction for SOD patients.

As such, SOD patients are suffering. In my opinion, the doctors who say they don't believe SOD is a real disorder say so because they can't find a cure or reliable treatment and are frustrated. Everyone is stumped, to say the least and it is easier to brush these patients aside than tackle such a complex issue. Even so, it is impossible to claim after several decades of solid research and patient experiences that SOD is not a valid condition—that this constellation of symptoms does not originate from the sphincter area. It is impossible to argue that every single biliary roux en y patient I've met no longer has that right side SOD pain because their sphincter of Oddi has been removed. And what about the study that isolated biopsies of sphincters from transduodenal sphincteroplasty surgeries? The one that proved 60% of specimens had physical signs of inflammation and fibrosis.

Delivering the Wrong Message about SOD

Researchers and doctors have been getting more than enough press and speaking opportunities to loudly refute SOD's existence. However, not one medical journal, symposium, or medical conference in recent years has bothered to capture the actual patient perspective or publish anything demanding innovative SOD research collaborating with or led by patients. Few of these outlets have published, in recent years, a single word about the decades of facts supporting SOD as a rebuttal to the SOD doubters. No one is reporting on the actual plight of SOD patients.

A perfect example of how blatantly irresponsible the medical community is with regard to SOD patients is an article published a few years ago in the American Gastroenterological Association's *Gastroenterology* journal titled, "Endoscopic Sphincterotomy for Sphincter of Oddi Dysfunction: Inefficacious Therapy for a Fictitious Disease." It was as if the authors and the journal's editors framed the article's title to deliberately sensationalize the topic to the detriment of patients everywhere. I wrote an op-ed piece responding to it on behalf of patients and the SODAE Network. Nearly two years ago, I was assured by the editor it would be published. I am yet to receive proof it was.

Can you imagine if the majority of medical articles written about prostate problems and breast cancer alluded to the fact these conditions were completely fictitious? These articles wouldn't get much play because it wouldn't be tolerated and neither should articles like this one about SOD. It should have never been published.

This opinion that SOD no longer exists is based on the fact the treatment at the center of the EPISOD study did not relieve symptoms in most participants and that a sham/placebo treatment fared better statistically—not that SOD could not diagnostically be proven. That treatment was the sphincterotomy. Theoretically, the authors claimed if the treatment did not relieve the patient's symptoms, then the problem could not have originated in the sphincter. This makes absolutely no sense. Would we say other diseases measured by symptomology and only slightly abnormal bloodwork or scans do not exist when a treatment is found to be ineffective, i.e. certain cancers, multiple sclerosis, Alzheimer's, etc.?

Researchers and medical professionals could instead do the right thing by SOD patients and postulate arguments for why this is happening and demand more research. As we know, many diseases cause secondary conditions. It is quite possible SOD began as a primary condition, but as it precipitated (it often takes years to obtain a diagnosis), it spawned secondary issues like ductal spasms, nerve and/or visceral hypersensitivity, malnutrition, or gut dysmotility. The original disease did not change. It was always there. However, once the sphincters were cut, the body still had these secondary issues, still tried to spasm, which continued to trigger pain. It makes total sense SOD patients still have pain after the sphincter is cut.

I am grateful I recovered from SOD and was well enough to write this book. I can finally tell the patient's story about the reality of SOD and what is happening to SOD patients. I am sick of hearing stories in our support group—all from women—about their doctors suddenly telling them they have IBS, a nerve problem, or a psychiatric issue after they were successfully treated for SOD for years, some for decades.

SOD Patients Abandoned and Misdiagnosed

There are too many examples of horrible things happening to SOD patients, I could fill an entire book with these accounts. One particular SOD patient had a successful sphincterotomy every year. After performing the sphincterotomy the doctor would comment to her on how tight her sphincter area was to the point he could barely get instruments in and that she always had signs of scar tissue. This same woman recently saw her doctor for a routine follow-up. She told us that no sooner did the doctor enter the exam room than he told her she would not get another sphincterotomy from him, ever; and that she did not have SOD.

He told her she had IBS (as far as I'm concerned, in this case, IBS stands for It's BullS—t). This woman needed a repeated sphincterotomy because her pressures were so high her papilla would get stenosis and scar tissue accumulated (as noted in her chart). She was baffled by his sudden change in demeanor and beside herself as she could not find another SOD doctor nearby who took her insurance. In addition, she could not afford to travel to another SOD specialist.

Another woman's doctor refused to continue placing stents that alleviated her pain and nausea. Last I heard she was on the verge of losing her job as she missed too much work from the flare ups. When she was getting the stents she never missed a day. These flare-ups were controlled by the stents. What is the big deal to not treat this poor woman?

Another woman had been doctor-less for two years because the only SOD doctor within driving distance who accepted her insurance no longer believed in SOD. Before this, she was getting balloon dilatations, stents, and antispasmodics. She had a good career during that time and was active in her children's extracurricular activities. Now she cannot work, is disabled, and cannot parent her children full time. Her mother is helping raise her children. All because no doctor will help her within her insurance limits.

Two women I have been helping via email had all of the hallmark SOD symptoms. Their test results were only slightly abnormal so no doctor near them would consider treating them for SOD. Both traveled to see SOD doctors from the SODAE Network doctor list and are now doing well from treatments. These women and those mentioned previously had SOD Type 2 or 3 and high manometric pressures.

I find it ironic that a largely female-dominant disease is trying to be abolished by an all-male faction of specialists yet not a single one is moving toward trying to understand why this disease affects women the most, i.e. by conducting hormonal and endocrine research. As patients, we need to band together because the situation is not getting better. It is getting worse. As I said, much of this is because of the EPISOD study interpretations. I was one of the test subjects for the study and there were more holes in it than a sieve.

The EPISOD Study: Warts and All

In May 2014, the much-anticipated results of the EPISOD study were described in a *Journal of the American Medical Association* article, "Effect of Endoscopic Sphincterotomy for Suspected Sphincter of Oddi Dysfunction on Pain-Related Disability Following Cholecystectomy: The EPISOD Randomized Clinical Trial." It was no surprise the results showed that SOD Type 3 patients did not gain relief from an ERCP with sphincterotomy versus a sham placebo group. I say "no surprise" because as I stated in Chapter 9, studies prior to this study revealed sphincterotomy is not an effective or reliable treatment for Type 3 patients and only beneficial to Type 2 patients with elevated manometry results. Therefore, we don't really know anything more than we knew prior to having millions of our U.S. tax dollars spent on this study.

What did surprise my fellow SOD sufferers and me was the way in which some researchers and doctors decided to use this study as a platform to say SOD was a fictitious disease. This "throw the baby out with the bath water" mentality angered pretty much all of us afflicted with this horrid condition. Most disappointing was not a single gastroenterologist who wrote about this study made a point to say we desperately need funding to figure out the causes of and treatments for SOD, particularly the overwhelmingly female prevalence. I am talking about studying real treatments like hormones, natural treatments, medications (not just antidepressants), Botox, and stop wasting our time on the anatomy of the sphincter and slicing it up.

Very few doctors are advocating for the SOD patient, but thank you to the few who *are* advocating for us and continuing to treat us. Though I am bashing a few doctors here, I need to make a point of expressing my gratitude to the doctors, most of whom are listed on the SODAE Network website, who have not waivered in their devotion and compassion toward SOD patients. Thank you. Thank you. Thank you. Your dedication has not gone unnoticed.

Unfortunately, in my opinion, there has been almost no compassion exhibited in commentaries written on this study in regard to SOD patients. No one has said, "Let's get to the bottom of this condition. These patients are suffering horribly and need a cure. Let's join together with patients and figure out why this condition exists."

Nope, instead many are saying, "Let's get rid of SOD as a diagnosis." Point blank. As such, some doctors have taken this as a green light to abandon patients or give patients a new, oftentimes false diagnosis. I have had to remove several SOD doctors from the SODAE Network SOD doctor list. Therefore, if you are wondering why a so-called SOD doctor is not on our list, chances are they were removed due to multiple patient complaints. It is unlikely we missed adding a good SOD doctor to the list unless the doctor is new to the SOD game or practices on a small scale.

Please contact us at the www.sodae.org website to request adding a recommended SOD doctor. It is quite telling that none of the doctors who have been removed from the list have ever been recommended again by any SOD patients.

In a perfect world, I would love nothing more than to see a former SOD doctor spend a week with an SOD patient. Take care of all the things, i.e. kids, laundry, groceries, cleaning, etc. which she cannot do because of SOD. Stab yourself in the side and feel the pain we feel (ok, maybe I'm going a bit far with that). Sit on a tilt-a-whirl ride at the county fair for 15 minutes and see how you feel. Imagine feeling that nauseous 24 hours a day, seven days a week. After they did all of these things, I would happily witness their report of how it all went.

Back to the EPISOD study. The EPISOD study's objective was to determine whether endoscopic sphincterotomy reduced pain and whether sphincter manometric pressure is predictive of pain relief. No other symptomology other than pain was measured, which was a huge issue for me. When my SOD became disabling, my right side pain took a backseat to horrible nausea, food sensitivities, pancreatic symptoms, and weight loss. It would have been nice if they measured patients' other symptoms.

I know many with SOD who get a sphincterotomy to relieve severe nausea and it worked. They could have cared less about pain. In fact, for two years in a row, The SODAE Network's patient surveys revealed SOD patients suffered from nausea more than pain. Like I said earlier, even if the sphincter area was cut, the entire muscle can still spasm, causing pain. That is a no-brainer. It would have been nice if other symptoms were measured, not just pain.

Patients were studied at seven different SOD specialty clinic centers. All patients had an ERCP but some got a sphincterotomy and some did not (sham). Patients did not know which category they fell into. After ERCP, patients were randomized 2:1 to sphincterotomy (n = 141) or sham (n = 73) irrespective of manometry findings. The Hogan-Geenen sphincter of Oddi classification proved there was a wide variation in sphincterotomy success with normal or abnormal manometry. Who had abnormal manometry? 64% had elevated biliary and pancreatic sphincters. 12% biliary alone.

I personally don't think anyone with normal manometry should have been included since manometry has already been proven to be the gold standard for diagnosing SOD. In my opinion, manometry is a good tool. But, of course, it was part of the study's objective goal, so they had to include low manometry scores. Those randomized to sphincterotomy with elevated pancreatic sphincter pressures were randomized again (1:1) to biliary or to both biliary and pancreatic sphincterotomies. Seventy-two were entered into an observational study with conventional ERCP management (this is the group I was in).

The results were lackluster. Twenty-seven patients (37%) in the sham treatment group versus 32 (23%) in the sphincterotomy group experienced successful treatment. Of the patients with pancreatic sphincter hypertension, 14 (30%) who underwent dual sphincterotomy and 10 (20%) who underwent biliary sphincterotomy alone experienced successful treatment. No clinical subgroups appeared to benefit from sphincterotomy more than others. Of the nonrandomized patients in the observational study group, 5 (24%) who underwent biliary sphincterotomy, 12 (31%) who underwent dual sphincterotomy, and 2 (17%) who did not undergo sphincterotomy had successful treatment.

The researchers concluded, "In patients with abdominal pain after cholecystectomy undergoing ERCP with manometry, sphincterotomy versus sham did not reduce disability due to pain. These findings do not support ERCP and sphincterotomy for these patients." Like I said before, I agree with the outcomes in so far as sphincterotomy doesn't work for SOD Type 3 pain. Again, what about nausea, weight loss, and other SOD symptoms? We don't know. Regardless, we do need to look to other treatments for this population. ERCP can be dangerous if you end up with acute pancreatitis. I nearly died from it. So, I am not a huge advocate of sphincterotomy or ERCP unless you have SOD Type 1 or 2.

Though I agreed with the outcomes, I think it is important I share about my experience as an EPISOD test subject, primarily the flaws.

I had a transduodenal sphincteroplasty three months after the dual sphincterotomy and yet the interviewers continued to include me in their follow-up screenings. I would inform them every time they'd call that I had this operation and they said it didn't matter. I would think I should have been disqualified sooner, but that may not have been an option for the NIH requirements. Whatever the excuse, I think my surgery should have been highlighted in the outcomes.

At each follow-up interview, the interviewer asked if I still had pain. She asked if I had abdominal pain, not SOD-specific pain, just "abdominal pain." At every six month follow-up I would say, "Yes." However, the abdominal pain was not SOD pain, it was pancreatic pain from my chronic pancreatitis. They were two different types of pain. Someone could have had a successful sphincterotomy yet continued to have pain in their abdomen from any number of conditions related to SOD or not. Not clarifying this with patients was a huge red flag in my opinion. I know SOD patients with chronic pancreatitis like me. Some have pain from ulcerative colitis, gastroparesis, IBS (the real IBS), scar adhesions, etc.

After I reviewed my medical records for the ERCP and dual sphincterotomy, I strongly suspected I was pushed into the Type 3 category to become eligible for the study. I was a perfect match for the study otherwise—no narcotic drug use or psychological problems, and normal scans/bloodwork. I am not accusing anyone of doing anything dishonest. I just find it odd that I missed being categorized SOD Type 2 by 1mm. I recently read more about the study and it turned out they were supposed to remove patients with bile ducts larger than 9mm in diameter. My ERCP report for the purposes of the study stated my bile duct was "11mm." I am still confused how I qualified.

I was on a benzodiazepine, clonazepam, and I firmly believe benzos contributed to some of my lingering SOD symptoms. It seemed the only medication of concern for EPISOD was narcotic pain medication. What if someone started on an antispasmodic, a muscle relaxer, or went off a medication that contributed to the sham getting relief? We will never know.

The interviewer did not ask if my diet had changed or if I began employing alternative treatment methods, all of which could have contributed to the success or failure of symptom relief.

Gender differences should have been a special component of this study, considering the high prevalence of female SOD patients. This was a very disappointing missed opportunity for research into the treatment success of women versus men.

Determining the final outcome of treatment success at months 9 and 12 was not a good choice. It is very common for the SOD patients I know to have a reoccurrence of symptoms due to stenosis and scar tissue formation at six or more months post-ERCP. Follow-up results should have been gauged at fewer months.

Researchers/Doctors Ignore SOD Patients' Reality

Recently I came across an article called, "Sphincter of Oddi Dysfunction Still Alive?" in the *American Gastroenterological Association*. The author, an EPISOD doctor and researcher, confessed his frustrations about this elusive condition and how he has gone to the side of SOD naysayers, especially after the completion of the EPISOD study.

He wrote, "Since SOD type III does not exist, and many Type I patients have an organic explanation that can be revealed by EUS, it is time to ditch the old I, II, III classification. We are left with one problem syndrome called "suspected SOD," whose complexities and components will be revealed gradually by further research."

I don't know about any of you, but I for one don't ever want a disease with the word "suspected" in it. That screams, "it's all in your head." I also don't agree he can say SOD 3 is dead. He also says, "this is the end of an era," as if we have to accept disposing of SOD because he says so. "Hey SOD doctors, drop your patients now." Although the author's intent may not be this, this is how many doctors are interpreting it.

He also complained in the article that he never accurately knew how his patients did once they left his center (many came from all over the country to get treatment yet never returned). He and all of the EPISOD researchers (he clearly says "we") concluded that most if not all of the "successes" in the study were due to a powerful placebo effect in very distressed patients coming to known "experts" and supported for a year by contact with research staff.

What is happening at the real-life ground level with patients is not what is imagined in cases like this. I cannot say there aren't patients who fall into this star struck placebo effect category he talks about. I have just never met one of them. Clearly, if this is the school of thought of most GI doctors, then they desperately need to visit an SOD support group and find out what is factual rather than forming opinions and assumptions.

First, not for a single moment did I ever feel being interviewed for this study was therapeutic. In fact, it was an annoyance. I did get a gift card, though, so I almost felt compelled to exaggerate how well I was doing as a thank you. Second, here are the reasons why I never made it back to the superstar expert SOD center: 1. I had the transduodenal sphincteroplasty three months after the EPISOD ERCP, which led me to feel better. 2. My insurance changed and I could not see an out of state doctor. There was no EPISOD center in my state. 3. No matter how bad my symptoms were I refused to ever get another ERCP again due to the near-death acute pancreatitis and E-coli sepsis infection I got at this stellar center.

I queried other EPISOD study test subjects from our support group. Here are some of the real life reasons why patients did not return to other EPISOD centers:

Patient 1 said, "I went to (the center) for the ERCP. After having acute pancreatitis, I was determined to never have another ERCP. I made a complete lifestyle change (diet-wise) and haven't had an ERCP since, hoping I never have to again. If I do I will go back, there. But it's 5 hours away." My note: I have watched this woman for the last three years via our support group. She drastically changed her diet after the EPISOD ERCP and, from my observation, has been in remission for this reason alone. She is strict and vigilant. She is a baker and won't even eat her own creations!

Patient 2 said, "I tried to go back to (the center) but was told they no longer treated SOD 3. Other women with SOD have heard the same thing from this center. I believe I had the sham and found someone local who has been treating me with medications that work."

Patient 3 said, "I lost my job from being sick too much. I also lost the insurance I had from my job that paid for the out-of-state doctor at (the center). I started feeling better after the ERCP I think because I didn't have the stress of a full-time job anymore and could focus on my health full-time. Now that I am back to work I am feeling sick again."

Patient 4 said, "I had a biliary roux en y not long after the EPISOD ERCP and feel great."

Much can be learned by simply taking the time to talk with patients or people working on the front lines advocating for these patients.

Nothing About Us Without Us

In the last article I mentioned, I agreed with this doctor's statement that it is time for a comprehensive reappraisal of "functional" biliary (and pancreatic) disorders. But patients *must* be included in the discussion and formulation of future research and diagnostic systems. Until that happens, any doctor or system removing SOD as a diagnosis should be liable for what happens to their patients. Any wrong-doing or patient abandonment should be treated as a human rights issue.

We cannot rely on the medical profession to "have our backs" after the backlash against patients following EPISOD. In any other field affecting consumers, patients are included as collaborators for the solution. Peer reviewers are required in research yet I have never met an SOD patient who has ever been involved in any review process as a peer and not a patient. The "nothing about us without us" theme occurring in other fields does not exist for SOD patients. It is time we change that. In other words, do not make a decision about our bodies without our input.

Rather than spending valuable time slamming SOD and changing the name, sufferers are in dire need for researchers, policymakers, and the medical profession as a whole to spearhead and fund research to identify the cause of this condition, which *does* occur in the sphincter of Oddi. By learning the exact nature and cause of SOD, we can then move on to identify and develop effective treatments and preventative measures.

I encourage you to get involved with SOD advocacy by visiting your elected officials, ex. Congressman, Senator, etc. to educate them on what it is like to have SOD. Get involved with groups like the SODAE Network or the International Foundation for Functional Gastrointestinal Disorders (www.iffgd.org).

Closing Statement

Thank you for taking the time to read this book. It was a labor of love that I hope will help you or someone you know with SOD. I wish you wellness and encourage you to get involved with SOD advocacy at www.sodae.org. Please visit my blog, Have a Healthy Gut, at www.haveahealthygut.com where I discuss a broad range of topics related to healthy digestion, including gut healing after gallbladder removal and antibiotics.

Bibliography

Adams, S. (2012, Apr 27). Why Do So Many Doctors Regret Their Job Choice? *Forbes*.

Al-Azzawi, A. (2012, Mar 18). Transduodenal Sphincteroplasty versus choledochoduodenostomy in management of lower common bile duct stones. *Basrah Journal Original Article of Surgery*.

Anderson, T. (1985, Apr). Experience with sphincteroplasty and sphincterotomy in pancreatobiliary surgery. *Annals of Surgery*. 201(4):399-406.

Bistritz, L. and Bain, V. (2006). Sphincter of Oddi dysfunction: Managing the patient with chronic biliary pain. *World Journal of Gastroenterology*. 12(24): 3793-3802.

Celiac Plexus Block. Ohio Health Member Hospitals. Retrieved from: http://www.medcentral.org/Main/CeliacPlexusBlock.aspx

Chan, H. (2011). Endoscopic Papillary Large Balloon Dilation Alone Without Sphincterotomy for the Treatment of Large Common Bile Duct Stones. *BMC Gastroenterology*.

Cholecystokinin. *Pathophysiology of the Digestive System*. Retrieved from: http://www.vivo.colostate.edu/hbooks/pathphys/endocrine/gi/cck.html

Cotton, P., et al. (2014, May). Effect of Endoscopic Sphincterotomy for Suspected Sphincter of Oddi Dysfunction on Pain-Related Disability Following Cholecystectomy: The EPISOD Randomized Clinical Trial. *JAMA*. 311(20):2101-2109.

Cotton, P. (2014, Sept). Sphincter of Oddi Dysfunction Still Alive? *American Gastroenterological Association*.

Digesting It All! *Connections: An Educational Resource for*

Women's International Pharmacy. Retrieved from: https://www.womensinternational.com/connections/digesting.html.

Drossman DA, Li Z, Andruzzi E, Temple RD, Talley NJ, Thompson WG, et al. (1993). U.S. householder survey of functional gastrointestinal disorders. Prevalence, sociodemography, and health impact. *Digestive Diseases and Sciences*. 38:1569-80.

Duca, S. (2003). Laparoscopic cholecystectomy: incidents and complications. A retrospective analysis of 9542 consecutive laparoscopic operations. *HPB : The Official Journal of the International Hepato Pancreato Biliary Association*. 5(3): 152–158.

EMDR Humanitarian Assistance Programs, Trauma Recovery Website. Retrieved from: http://www.emdrhap.org/content/what-is-emdr/

Endometriosis and Prostaglandins. Endometriosis Resolved Website. Retrieved from: http://www.endo-resolved.com/prostaglandins.html

Fuentes, A. (2012, May 24). "Men and Women Are the Same Species!". *Psychology Today*.

Goldman, L. (2011). *Goldman's Cecil Medicine* (24th ed.).

Greer J., Park E., Safren S. (2010 Jan 1). Tailoring Cognitive-Behavioral Therapy to Treat Anxiety Comorbid with Advanced Cancer. *Journal of Cognitive Psychotherapy*. 24(4): 294–313.

Hogan, W. (2007). Diagnosis and Treatment of Sphincter of Oddi Dysfunction. *Gastroenterology and Hepatology*. 3(1): 31–35.

Hormones, the Pancreas, and Obesity. *Discovery's Edge* (Mayo Clinic Magazine). Retrieved from: http://www.mayo.edu/research/discoverys-edge/hormones-pancreas-obesity

Kline, et al. (2005, Aug). "Progesterone inhibits gallbladder motility through multiple signaling pathways". *Steroids*. 70(9):673-9

Lee, S, et al. (2001, Feb). Electroacupuncture May Relax the Contraction of Sphincter of Oddi. *Gastrointestinal Endoscopy*. 53(2):211-6.

Levine, J. (2015, Jun). The Science of Breathing. *Yoga Journal*.

Liang T., et al. (2016, Mar). Roles of Sphincter of Oddi Laxity in Bile Duct Microenvironment in Patients with Cholangiolithiasis: From the Perspective of the Microbiome and Metabolome. *Journal of the American College of Surgery*. 222(3):269-280.e10.

Lingen, J. (2012, Mar). "The Second Trimester: Constipation, Gas, & Heartburn". *Healthline*.

Luman, W., et al. (1997). "Influence of Cholecystectomy on Sphincter of Oddi Motility". *Gut*. 41:371-374 doi:10.1136/gut.41.3.371.

McCammon, RL, et al. (1978, Jun). Effect of Transdermal Fentanyl Patches on the Motility of the Sphincter of Oddi. *Anesthesiology*. 48(6):437.

McLoughlin, MT and Mitchell, RMS. (2007 Dec). Sphincter of Oddi dysfunction and pancreatitis. *World Journal of Gastroenterology*. 13(47): 6333-6343

Mirza, M. (2014, June 25). Ginger Reduces Inflammation and Pain. Retrieved from: https://painpatient.com/2014/06/25/ginger-reduces-inflammation-and-pain/

Ravindra, KV. (1996). Choledochoduodenostomy: influence of risk factors in post-operative morbidity. *Indian Gastroenterology*. 15(1):4-6.

Relaxin. (2015, Mar). You and Your Hormones. *The Society for Endocrinology.*

Secretin. *Pathophysiology of the Digestive System.* Retrieved from: http://www.vivo.colostate.edu/hbooks/pathphys/endocrine/gi/secretin.html.

Sherman, S. and Lehman, G. (2001). Sphincter of Oddi Dysfunction: Diagnosis and Treatment. *Journal of the Pancreas.* 2(6):382-400.

Sherman, S. (1996, Sept). Effects of meperidine on the pancreatic and biliary sphincter. *Gastrointestinal Endoscopy.* 44(3):239–242.

Sherman, S., Tran, H. (2006 Feb). Pneumobilia: benign or life-threatening. *Journal of Emergency Medicine.* 30(2):147-53.

Spinal Cord Stimulation. Mayfield Brain and Spine Clinic. http://www.mayfieldclinic.com/PE-STIM.htm

Stinton, L. and Shaffer, E. (2012, Apr). "Epidemiology of Gallbladder Disease: Cholelithiasis and Cancer". *Gut Liver.* 6(2): 172–187.

Tantia O., Jain M., Khanna S., Sen B. (2008 Jul-Sep). Post cholecystectomy syndrome: Role of cystic duct stump and re-intervention by laparoscopic surgery. *Journal of Minimal Access Surgery.* 4(3): 71–75.

The surprising dangers of CT scans and X-rays. (2015, Jan 15). *Consumer Reports.*

Tierney, S., et al. (1994, Jul). Estrogen inhibits sphincter of Oddi motility". *The Journal of Surgical Research.* 57(1):69-73.

Tierney, S., et al. (1999, Feb). "Progesterone alters biliary flow dynamics". *Annals of Surgery.* 229(2): 205–209.

Torrey, T. (2016, May 6). Complain About a Doctor or Other

Healthcare Provider. https://www.verywell.com/complain-about-a-doctor-or-other-healthcare-provider-2614928#step5.

Wehrmann T, Seifert H, Seipp M, Lembcke B, Caspary WF. (1998 Oct 30). Endoscopic injection of botulinum toxin for biliary sphincter of Oddi dysfunction.
Endoscopy. (8):702-7.

Wikipedia: Estrogen. https://en.wikipedia.org/wiki/Estrogen

Wikipedia: Ginger. https://en.wikipedia.org/wiki/Ginger

Zhang, ZH, et al. (2008 Jul 7). "Sphincter of Oddi hypomotility and its relationship with duodenal-biliary reflux, plasma motilin and serum gastrin". *World Journal of Gastroenterology*. 14(25):4077-81.

About the Author

Brooke Keefer is the proud mother of three sons, a stepdaughter, stepson, and has two grandchildren. Brooke has a Bachelor of Arts degree in Mathematics from the State University of New York at Albany. For over 15-years, she worked as a not-for-profit director, lobbyist, advocate, and wrote, managed and reviewed grants in the field of children's mental health and juvenile justice. Brooke has several disabling conditions including sphincter of Oddi dysfunction, chronic pancreatitis, and fluoroquinolone toxicity syndrome (caused by a long-term adverse reaction to the antibiotic Levaquin). She now dedicates her work to bringing awareness to these diseases, writing health articles, advocating for patient rights, and recently started a digestive health blog called Have a Healthy Gut at www.haveahealthygut.com. Brooke is the founder of the Sphincter of Oddi Dysfunction Awareness and Education Network, a 501c3 not for profit organization. She manages its website, www.sodae.org, and Facebook page and support group.

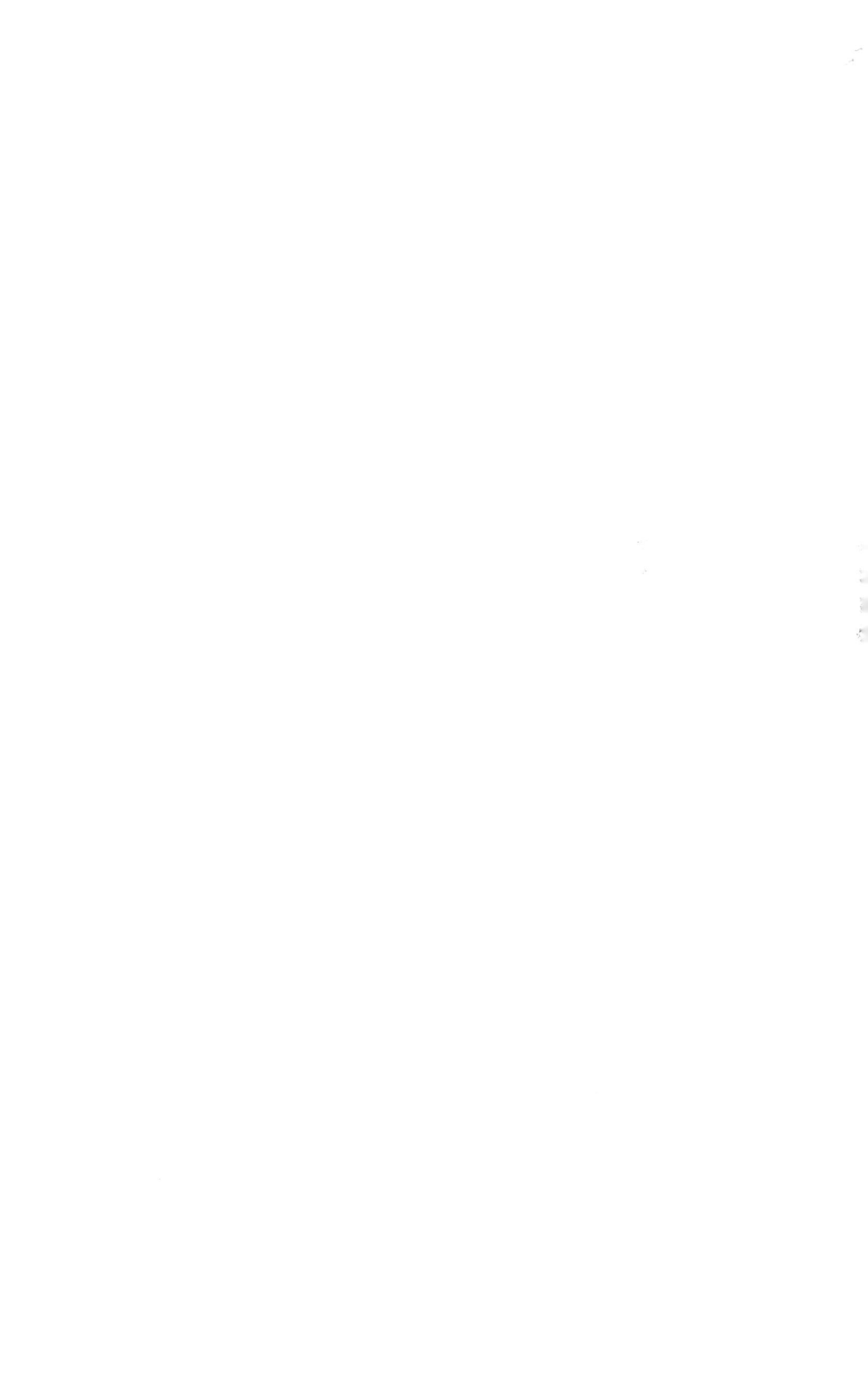

Made in the USA
Columbia, SC
12 December 2021